The Sino-American Friendship as Tradition and Challenge

The Sino-American Friendship as Tradition and Challenge

Dr. Ailie Gale in China, 1908–1950

M. Cristina Zaccarini

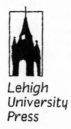

Lehigh
University
Press

Bethlehem: Lehigh University Press
London: Associated University Presses

Associated University Presses
440 Forsgate Drive
Cranbury, NJ 08512

Associated University Presses
16 Barter Street
London WC1A 2AH, England

Associated University Presses
P.O. Box 338, Port Credit
Mississauga, Ontario
Canada L5G 4L8

The paper used in this publication meets the requirements of the American National Standard for Permanence of Paper for Printed Library Materials Z39.48-1084.

Library of Congress Cataloging-in-Publication Data

Zaccarini, Maria Cristina.
    The Sino-American friendship as tradition and challenge : Dr. Ailie Gale in China, 1908–1950 / M. Cristina Zaccarini.
        p. cm.
    Includes bibliographical references and index.
    ISBN 0-934223-70-X (alk. paper)
    1. Gale, Ailie. 2. Missionaries, Medical—China—Biography. 3. Women physicians—China—Biography. 4. Women missionaries—China—Biography. 5. China—History—20th Century. I. Title.
R722.32.G35 Z33 2001
610'.92—dc21
B   00-066281

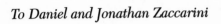

To Daniel and Jonathan Zaccarini

Contents

Preface

While the Chinese government has expressed preference for Pinyin, I have used the Wade-Giles system because this is the romanization that the missionaries used.

Acknowledgments

This study was begun at the history department of the State University of Stony Brook, under the direction of my advisor, Dr. Michael Barnhart, who inspired me to want to learn more about how missionaries contributed to public perceptions of a "Sino-American friendship." Dr. Barnhart's patience, and his insistence on clarity and precise writing, guided me to the end of the dissertation process. Members of my doctoral dissertation committee, Dr. Bill Miller and Dr. Nancy Tomes offered critiques that enabled me to reevaluate my work.

Dr. John L. Rawlinson read my early work, offering not only scholarly assistance, but also a unique glimpse into the life experience and memories of a son of missionaries. John L. Rawlinson continues to be an important source of support for me. Dr. Kathleen Lodwick, another committee member, taught me much about the complexities of twentieth-century China. Kathleen Lodwick has continued to follow the progress of my work and remains a very generous and helpful friend. Dr. Randi Warne, a scholar and friend, gave me courage and support at critical stages of my research. While I owe everyone who inspired, critiqued and supported me a heartfelt thank you, I must absolve them of any errors or omissions that remain in this book.

At the early stages of my research I came to benefit from the help and insights of Hilah Thomas, historian and consultant for the Women's Division, Board of Global Ministries Oral History Project. I am grateful to Ms. Thomas for allowing me to use some of her rich sources. At the General Board of Global Ministries I enjoyed several interesting discussions about women missionaries over lunch with Hilah Thomas, Bud Carroll and Diane Allen, all of whom were immensely helpful and supportive.

I am thankful for the time, consideration and attention given to me by former missionaries and friends of the Gale family. In particular, Hilda Weiss Andrus, Louise Cate, Joel Johnson, Carrel Morgan and Phoebe White Wentworth, Shanghai American School Historian, were most helpful with recollections, interviews and letters.

11

Parts of this manuscript were first delivered at a Research Forum of the North Atlantic Missiology Project in Pasadena in March 1998, coordinated by the University of Cambridge and financed by The Pew Charitable Trusts. While I gratefully acknowledge the support of the Trusts, the opinions expressed here are mine and do not necessarily reflect their views. I am grateful to Dr. Brian Stanley, for his advice and encouragement at the forum, and to Dr. Dana Robert and Dr. Ralph Elphick for their helpful suggestions.

Without the assistance of archivists at the following libraries, this project would have been impossible; I would like to thank Joan Duffy at theYale Divinity School library, Patrick Gilbo, at the American Red Cross National Headquarters, Ernest Rubinstein, of the Ecumenical Library, Interchurch Center, Tom Rosenbaum and Anke Voss-Hubbard, of the Rockefeller Archives Center, Mark Shenise and Dale Patterson at Drew University, the Archives of the United Methodist Church, Sharon Abbey at Lane Medical Library Archives and Special Collections, Ginny Kiefer of the Tutt Library, Colorado College, William J. Walsh, at the National Archives and Records Administration at College Park, Betty Clements, of the Claremont School of Theology, Victor Oliva, Trudy Neubaur and Sheila Salamon at the Adelphi University library and Shelter Rock library's C-El Purdy.

I am thankful to the late Dr. Frank C. Gale, Jr., who generously provided me with the correspondence of his mother, Dr. Ailie Gale and for the invaluable assistance of Hildur Gale. Mrs. Gale kept her husband's memories alive with her loving attentiveness. I reaped the benefit of this when, during our many long telephone conversations, Frank Gale shared with me these vivid stories of his mother. Many thanks to members of the Gale family who contacted me after hearing of my work on Ailie Gale, offering further valuable anecdotes and sources.

While in the final stages of revision of this manuscript, I have been fortunate to have had the privilege of working with exceptional scholars and educators at the History Department of Adelphi University. To professors Marty Haas and Patrick Kelly in particular, I wish to express my gratitude for years of encouragement, inspiration and friendship that I will treasure forever.

Above all, I'm grateful to my husband Juan and my parents for their love and support, without which I could not have researched or written anything.

Introduction

GLOBAL INTERDEPENDENCE AND THE INTERNATIONAL CRISES OF our time cry out for a better understanding of the forging of transnational ties and the shaping of public opinion in our nation's history. An especially instructive point of focus for scholars are the twentieth-century American public's feelings of sentimental friendship toward China, a country in which American cultural, economic and political interests continue to converge.

The American public's mood was an essential aspect of the climate within which foreign policy decision-making took place during the first half of the twentieth century.[1] The public's sentimental attitude toward China played a part in the Franklin D. Roosevelt administration's considerations regarding the United States' Asian policy during the 1930s and 1940s.[2] By the time the Roosevelt administration's New Deal focus shifted to an internationalist outlook in 1941, requiring the American public's support for China, the seeds of friendship had already been sown by missionaries.

Scholars have sought to explain American perceptions of friendship with China by exploring the vast literature produced by male missionaries in visible positions of administrative power.[3] However, the writings of an important segment of public opinion shapers, the missionary movement's female majority, remain unexamined.

Walking into missionary society meetings in 1930, one man in the Middle Western United States reported feeling as though he had "dropped by mistake into a secret society whose lingo" he could not understand. At a 1944 Foreign Missions Conference a male speaker identified the reason for the unfamiliar "lingo" when he reported: women, rather than men, were "familiar with the missionary movement."[4] Indeed, the movement appealed largely to American women because women comprised over 60 percent of the missionary force. I believe that the American public's sentimental attitude toward China was, in significant part, a product of women missionaries' images of that nation as

13

a nurturing ground for ideals which were appealing to many Protestant women.[5]

This book examines the "lingo" of the missionary movement to understand the assumptions of its members, which I term a presumed "sisterhood" of Protestant women. Because the broad and complex problems I address here require a manageable point of focus, my emphasis, for the twentieth-century portion of this work, will only be on the cultural and social milieu and correspondence of one woman missionary, Dr. Ailie Gale, a member of the Methodist Episcopal Church North, the most representative denomination in America until the mid-twentieth century.

As historian Nathan O. Hatch has observed, the Methodists were the most "quintessentially American" of all denominations. From their eighteenth-century beginnings, the number of Methodist adherents had risen, outstripping much older and established Protestant denominations. From 1840 to the mid-twentieth century, they were the largest religious group in Protestant America, numbering 5.7 million in 1906 and over 8 million in about 40,000 congregations in 1946.[6]

The Methodists were a force to be reckoned with in China. Their worldwide missionary organization had begun work there in 1847, and by the twentieth century the Methodist Episcopal Church had one of the largest Protestant missions in China.[7] From 1921 to 1941, for example, the Methodist Episcopal Board of Foreign Missions (MEBFM) and their woman's board, the Women's Foreign Missionary Society (WFMS) sent more than 700 missionaries to China. During those years the numbers of missionaries ranged from 254 to 588.[8]

From 1911 to 1949, the numbers of married and single Methodist women dominated those of their male counterparts in every mission area of China. For example, of the total 309 missionaries in China throughout 1911, only 99 were men. That year the MEBFM's 94 women and the WFMS's 116 single women outnumbered their male counterparts in the following areas: Foochow, 54 women and 24 men; Hinghwa, 18 and 6; Central China, 48 and 22; North China, 51 and 28; and West China, 39 and 19. By 1920 the missionary force was 371: 261 women and 110 men. Of the 261 women, 169 were single and working either for the WFMS or MEBFM, and 92 were married.[9]

Women missionaries corresponded with American mission supporters from their posts in Southwest, Central, West and North China to encourage contributions to the China mission field. The success of missionaries' appeals depended upon their success at cultivating a relationship with their American supporters, as well as their skill at presenting appealing images of their work in China.[10]

I examine the self-representation of medical missionary Ailie Gale within the context of American supporters' presumed perception of women's status and roles in the United States and particularly in the American medical field. In so doing, I illuminate an important aspect of the values that underlay the American female public's perception of a special Sino-American friendship.

It was because she was a privileged white woman that Gale could pose some challenges to American middle-class perceptions of the proper role of women.[11] I examine the process by which Gale acquired home field funds, thus shedding light upon the larger issue of how American women missionaries benefited from the privileges associated with their status as Westerners. One important thesis presented here is that Gale's acquisition of supporter monies stemmed from her ability to function as a spokesperson for both novel and traditional perspectives, and by addressing, what historian Fred Weinstein describes as the "heterogeneous strivings (cognitive, moral and wishful)" of home field supporters.[12] Proceeding from the recognition that privileged white women do not fit neatly into one category, I present Gale as one type of woman who drew upon nineteenth-century assumptions, meanings and strivings that were appealing to some Methodist women while simultaneously challenging some conceptions of the proper role of women in the twentieth century.

Like many of her female contemporaries, when Gale arrived in Nanchang, Kiangsi, she did not openly declare herself imbued with the desire to lead or thrill gaping crowds, "whip" the world or "uplift" a civilization in "chains," as historian Xi Lian has observed of many male missionaries.[13] Conversely, Gale was not a formerly restricted churchwoman, liberated from Victorian gender restrictions by her relocation to China. Rather, Gale's self-representation as a successful doctor and administrator was an extension of an aspect of nineteenth-century American female Protestant culture that had enabled some women to achieve what I term empowerment-through-piety. Gale's interpretation of Christianity had given her the confidence to speak and take leadership roles within the church setting in the United States at the turn-of-the-century. Gale's confidence stemmed from an aspect of nineteenth-century American female culture which is often unacknowledged due to secular feminist scholars' need to maintain practical categories of analysis.

According to Nancy Cott, feminism was born in the 1910s, with the denial that men and women were different in any but the biological way.[14] Gale's writing style and content predates this definition in its consistency with the values of many nineteenth-century women missionaries.

Despite this, Nancy Cott's three components for defining a "feminist" are useful for understanding the bond between Gale and home field supporters. The first is a woman's awareness of belonging to a female social grouping, and the consequent realization "that one's experience reflects and affects the whole." Secondly, Cott describes a feminist as one who does *not* believe her group's condition to be "predestined by God or nature," because Cott believes that this belief would preclude a woman from perceiving any possible changes to her position. Lastly, to be considered "feminist" one must be in "opposition to sex hierarchy."[15]

I believe that before the term "feminist" came to be, the "sisters," a group comprised of missionaries and those involved with missionary work, not only perceived themselves as a woman's group but also behaved in a manner that reflected opposition to sex hierarchy. They did so on the basis of a God-centeredness that Cott identifies as repugnant to feminism: Protestant tenets and the obligations arising from them. Consequently, this study suggests that the nineteenth-century "sisters" who preceded Gale may not have been conscious or overt "feminists," but many spoke in a language which advocated an increased role for women, justified by piety.

In part 1, chapter 1 illustrates how married and single women created women's missionary societies while conscious of their unique status as women in opposition to male-dictated Victorian notions of separate spheres for men and women. Communication among Northern and Southern sisters led to their imitation of strategies and implementation of ideas for furthering the missionary cause. While Cott's definition renders feminism and religiosity mutually exclusive, I hope to illustrate that by believing in female and male spiritual equality and a woman's duty to serve God and humanity, the sisters could often erase social and regional disparities and bind together as a cohesive group, conscious of their special womanly struggles and of an existing gender discrimination and sex hierarchy that they must work against.

Common conceptions of piety allowed women to redefine their public place and to expand the parameters of female public speaking within the context of their efforts to raise money for the missionary cause. Chapter 1 illustrates how nineteenth-century American churchwomen organized missionary societies while conscious of the socially perceived incorrectness of their venture into the public sphere to raise monies. I argue that they were aware that men were responsible for controlling their opportunity to engage in the activities that required their presence in places that were deemed not befitting a woman, yet they defied these restrictions nonetheless.[16]

When churchwomen organized missionary societies and engaged in fund-raising activities they justified their actions by describing their prayers and communication with God or the Holy Spirit. In so doing, the women engaging in missionary work used the power of God to oppose and supplant the power of men.[17] While this did not mean that they wanted complete equality with men, the sisters believed that a divine calling would augment rather than limit, their place in society.

An outgrowth of this shared belief in the meaning of piety, was the "female-cultivation-through piety" ideal, which offered a view of women's education that contrasted with the prevailing consensus among Victorians. In chapters 2 and 3 I examine how nineteenth-century sisters educated themselves beyond what was deemed necessary by Victorian culture, thus defying another male-imposed restriction.[18] Declaring that education would allow them to better serve God and humanity, the women were chronicled in classic missionary literature as having gone on to overcome extraordinary practical and physical obstacles to educate themselves and enter the medical profession.

Chapter 2 illustrates that during the late nineteenth century, a period when female doctors opened women's medical schools and struggled to attain legitimacy in the newly emerging field of medicine in America, Methodist publications portraying women missionary physicians as competent professionals gave their American sisters support. In so doing, I believe that the literature addressed churchwomen supporters' wishful strivings and that these helped strengthen the bond between missionaries and the home field. Male critics of women in the professions argued that females were weak, prone to illness and physically unable to perform as men's professional equals.[19] Conversely, women physicians in the mission field told supporters of long, exhaustive hours of complex medical duties, including surgery, and the admiration of their male Western colleagues and the Chinese of all classes, thus challenging male representations of women's physical and professional inferiority. Consequently, we can view women medical missionaries' confident assertions, as expressed in Methodist literature, as a subversion of Victorian notions of women's physical weakness and professional inadequacy.

When nineteenth-century society, with its emphasis upon "germ theory," increasingly came to undervalue the soft and nurturing sides of healing typically associated with women, women missionaries' representation challenged this loss of value. As I illustrate in chapter 2, nineteenth-century medical women challenged the presumed superiority of men by questioning the superiority of the scientific areas of medicine which emphasized the disease, rather than the patient.

As scholars have noted, cultural superiority and Westerners' awareness of the germ theory of disease prompted women missionaries to portray the Chinese as unclean in opposition to Western cleanliness. Moreover, women doctors would express disdain for the popular stream of Chinese medicine that emphasized shamans, acupuncturists and soothsayers.[20]

Despite this reality, female doctors in China often benefited from the fact that their values mirrored important Confucian and Taoist dimensions of Chinese medicine. Women doctors in America had been valued for humaneness and compassion, and identified with a traditional approach to medicine that explained sickness as a condition affecting the entire organism. The medical training of women mirrored the Confucian emphasis upon humanity and compassion in medicine and Taoist pursuits of the harmonious integration of human and social elements. Hence, there was an affinity between those qualities associated with the practices and talents of women doctors—increasingly rejected by proponents of pure, objective science—and certain Confucian and Taoist dimensions of Chinese medicine. When women missionaries reported that officials and upper-class Chinese provided validation for women medical missionary doctors' efforts, they linked China to those aspects of American culture valued by American churchwomen. This linkage not only provided validation for traditional women's values but also inadvertently challenged the notion of Chinese inferiority.

The validation of the Chinese became especially important in the twentieth century. The Progressive era saw the emergence of professions that mirrored what Americans viewed as feminine concerns, or woman's work. During this era, public health became institutionalized but its leaders would be male, rather than female and its emphases would be on scientific concerns. Soon mainstream Americans manifested a declining concern with the humanistic, holistic medical interests that had flourished during the heyday of the Progressive movement. During this post-Progressive, post-World War I period, a new hero, the medical scientist, or the physician who valued technical skills over preventative medicine, gained the admiration of the male-dominated medical profession.[21] Women medical missionaries who portrayed themselves as successful in China provided validation for the feminized, humanistic medicine which had fallen into disfavor among many male doctors in the United States. As such, they continued the legacy of representing China as a nurturing ground for the humanistic medicine associated with women.

Part 2 of this book illustrates how Gale continued the legacy of her nineteenth-century sisters through her self-representation as a competent professional. Gale would tell supporters of successful public health programs implemented with the assistance and recognition of Chinese supporters. She would describe Chinese patients' willingness to accept and implement her public health policies, and Chinese officials' expressions of honor for her public health work throughout her years in

China. Chapter 6 illustrates how Gale depicts Chiang Kai-shek's New Life Program as complementary to her own and many women doctors' concerns and efforts in public health. Moreover, Gale described her adopted Chinese daughter Mary's growing affinity for public health nursing. Gale tried to make supporters feel as though their monies and letters were an important component to all of the successes she described in the field of public health.

These achievements validated humanistic medicine—a traditional female approach—while others suggested a direct challenge to assumptions of male superiority in the medical field. By the time Gale arrived in the China field in 1908, the position of women in the American medical field had deteriorated significantly. Nearly all the women's medical schools established in the nineteenth century had closed. As the numbers of women medical students and doctors declined and internships were rendered inaccessible to them, the accomplishments of women like Gale provided readers with a view of a successful woman doctor who excelled in areas that the American medical field normally considered within the male domain.

Much of Gale's success was in defiance of traditional views premised upon the superiority of not only male values, but the superiority of men in the medical field. Gale would serve as a hospital superintendent and administrator, design the blueprints for the reconstruction of hospitals and additions to medical buildings, create a hospital where none existed, using supporter funds and no assistance from the Methodist Episcopal Board, and describe performing complex surgeries. These activities were common for women medical missionaries in the China field, and doubtlessly, a major component of perceptions of a Sino-American friendship at this time was owed to the fact that women missionaries helped make them the common knowledge of American home field supporters.[22]

Given Gale's credibility with supporters, some evinced the view that she was a good source for learning more about China's political developments. In this capacity as well, Gale continued the legacy of her nineteenth-century sisters. The sisters' desire to propagate knowledge of foreign lands had originated with the early formation of women's missionary societies, and their emphasis upon educating members regarding other countries' cultures and their women. The ideal's emphasis upon concern for "heathen" women was truly a reflection of Western arrogance, yet it had enabled the "sisters" to raise money for the missionary cause, send women doctors to the foreign field and envision a cosmopolitan female role, where interests expanded from the household to the world.[23] These interests sustained traditional views of Western superiority, but they also threatened Victorian notions of separate spheres for men and women and the male-dictated conception that women's concerns remain at the domestic or national level rather than extend to the global realm.

Gale described the new Chinese Republic, the Nationalist movement, Chiang Kai-shek, the Sino-Japanese war and the Chinese Communists by focusing upon issues of importance to female home field supporters. One important aspect of this focus was Gale's interest in the place of women. Gale ignored the differences among Chinese and American women and issues of class, by comparing China to the United States, and linking China's political maturity and her acceptance of Christianity with the modernization and the empowerment of Chinese women.[24]

Beginning during the years after the 1911 revolution, Gale compared China's emerging nationhood to the United States in her Republican period. She reminded readers that their own nation's early years were fraught with problems, and that Christianity would resolve China's difficulties. Gale believed that with Chinese acceptance of Christian-educated Nationalist leaders, Chinese women would have more power and independence.

Gale correlated China's growing Nationalism with Chinese acceptance of Christianity and the corresponding improvements in the lives of Chinese women. In late 1911 Gale described the respect accorded to Chinese Christian-educated missionary doctor Ida Kahn and her hospital by Nationalist leader Dr. Sun Yat-sen and the city's populace and officials.[25] As Chinese Nationalism developed anti-Christian expressions during the 1920s, Gale was in Tunki, a rural mission station in Central China. Despite the anti-Christian demonstrations around her, Gale reported that she and her hospital were safe and protected and that Chinese women continued to benefit from the Nationalist presence in the area. By 1927, Gale emphasized not only that local and Nationalist leaders offered protection to missionaries and their property, but that Nationalists assigned places of honor to Christian Chinese women, helping to improve the Tunki populace's attitude toward the Methodist Church. Gale ignored the differences among Chinese and American women by suggesting that, just as Christianity had improved the lives of American women, through the vehicle of Nationalist victory, it would improve the lives of their Chinese sisters.

During her years in the Nationalist capital of Nanking, beginning in 1931, Gale increasingly came into contact with Nationalist leaders and a member of Chiang's inner circle of advisors, Protestant missionary George Shepherd. From this vantage point, she informed supporters of the Nationalist government's incorporation of public health policies. Gale's observations reflected the considerable resources Chiang devoted to control outbreaks of cholera, smallpox and plague. Moreover, since

preventative medicine was a traditionally female endeavor, Gale's touting
of Nationalist efforts had the effect of both linking Chiang's Nationalist
party to an area traditionally of concern to reform-minded Protestant
women and elevating China in the eyes of American churchwomen.[26]

Gale reiterated Nationalist officials' statements reflecting their conceptions of Chinese women as leaders in the reconstruction of China. She
told supporters that Christian China offered women new opportunities
that would obligate them to cultivate their minds and offer them equality
with men. Gale's descriptions of the opportunities available for Chinese
women mirrored the nineteenth-century ideal of "female cultivation-
through-piety." Gale's remarks suggested that in rapidly modernizing
China, where women's roles were changing, women missionary responses
had not been uniformly reactionary. Like many Methodist women, Gale
encouraged the Chinese women she knew, including her daughter, to
pursue careers so that their lives might be independent of male influence
and control.

As chapter 7 illustrates, Gale's perception of Nationalists' acceptance
of Christianity led her to interpret the Sino-Japanese conflict in both
gendered and religious terms. Gale's reports defied the typical binary
oppositions attributed to missionaries by most scholars as Japanese/strong
male versus Chinese/weak female. Gale depicted both the Chinese and
Japanese as strong, however, one represented Satan, and the other God.
Christian China was humanistic and thoughtful in her military actions,
while the Japanese military was devilish in its ruthlessness. Gale predicted
that eventually the Satanic Japanese military force would be wearied by
Christian China's growing retaliatory strength.

As the Nationalist government lost its appeal for supporters, Gale
understood Chinese desires for Communist victory. Chapter 9 explains
Gale's attitude toward Chinese Communism. Like most missionaries,
Gale objected to Communism because of its antagonism to Christian
religious services, and those female social programs which had been
the staple of the sisters' interest in China since the nineteenth century.
Gale described China's new Communist government in the context of
concerns and assumptions that she had emphasized in earlier writings.
She complained that Communist enthusiasts interfered with her medical
work and the ability of other missionaries to carry on their social programs.
Importantly, Gale objected to Communism's basic tenet, which required
equal work for each individual because she perceived it as discriminatory
for many needy Chinese, particularly single mothers with large families.

Gale's naïve perceptions of Chinese Nationalists, her inability to com-
prehend the import of the Chinese Communist victory, her lack of
criticism of Western imperialism and her cultural superiority suggest

that Gale was in many ways conservative. Yet, alongside this conservative perspectives were forces for challenge and change.

This study suggests that the effect of Gale's self-representation as a successful woman doctor challenged American home field supporters' prejudice against women in medicine. Due to the gradually decreasing numbers of women in medicine in the United States from 1910 to 1950, home field supporters had fewer opportunities to view a woman presenting herself as a competent professional doctor. Moreover, American women doctors were not commonly seen building and administering hospitals, or performing surgery, because they were mostly relegated to the fields of pediatrics and public health, traditionally female realms in which men held leadership positions.

Presenting Gale as a model for the expansion of women's roles away from conventional venues appears uncongenial in light of contemporary feminist historians' view that feminism is about the empowerment of all women and change in the conditions of all women's lives. As a white woman, doctor, administrator, surgeon and missionary, Gale's challenges to white male power may be viewed as empowering white women while simultaneously implying their superiority over Chinese women. Gale's self-representation as a successful administrator and her access to American supporters' contributions, a form of privilege unavailable to most Chinese women, replaced the notion of white male dominance with that of white privileged female dominance over the Chinese. Moreover, had Gale not posed a challenge to white patriarchal authority, her essential goal of supplanting Chinese culture with Western would still have been an unempowering one.

Conversely, to convict Gale for her elitism and support of traditional women's values that men deemed inferior, and that feminists rallied against, would deprive historians from understanding how women like Gale used these values to generate challenge. While Gale was elitist in her belief that she should supplant Chinese ways with Western, she simultaneously resisted many conceptions of American and Chinese women's inferior place. She both consciously and unconsciously used her status as a white medical doctor, with access to American funds, to challenge certain conceptions of the superiority of American culture, particularly as defined by male values.

Gale valued female interests such as "social concern," yet she did not assume that these were the direct result of biology, but culture. Projecting certain values, typically associated with women, as positive and powerful, Gale challenged male assertions of their lesser importance.

Gale's writings support Dana Robert's recent social history of American women in mission. Professor Robert identifies the shift from the sisterhood's emphasis upon "Woman's Work for Woman," to "World Friendship," which had as its basis, the belief that men and women could work together as equals through missions, for global issues of peace and justice, intertwined with the idea of improving conditions for women and children.[27] Gale's letters to supporters help shed light upon how this conception of "world friendship" was manifested during World War II, when, like many missionaries, Gale found that she could no longer promote pacifism. Gale's writings strongly support the view that twentieth-century women missionaries perceived themselves as having a global role, thereby suggesting that the existing scholarly consensus that early-twentieth-century women were relegated to national, and men to the global realm, requires reassessment. Gale's life and career shed light upon how some women missionaries, who embodied the seeds of both tradition and challenge, persuaded a segment of the American female public to forge transnational ties to the Chinese from 1911, the birth of the Chinese Republic, to 1949, the victory of the Chinese Communists and the climax to decades of struggle for national unity.[28]

The Sino-American
Friendship as Tradition
and Challenge

Part I

1

Women's Missionary Societies

IMAGES OF CHINA CREATED BY AILIE GALE IN THE EARLY TWEN-
tieth century were rooted in assumptions that were at the heart of the
community of Protestant women beginning in Victorian America. These
assumptions were central to the relationship that would develop between
Gale and her twentieth-century supporters in the home mission field.

While we cannot call them "values" because not all the women acted
upon them, these assumptions permitted many women to share a common language of Christian empowerment. The language facilitated bonds
between married and single women and its usage crossed social and
economic distinctions. The assumptions and language derived from an
interpretation of female piety that was shaped by the populist nature of
Methodism's influence on American culture and its women.

Classic nineteenth-century female Methodist missionary texts chronicle the instances where the product of female piety could counter
deeply entrenched cultural norms. The evolution of nineteenth-century
industrialization and the accompanying division between home and work
were reflected in a growing demarcation between the lives of men and
women. As the middle-class ideology of separate spheres increasingly
fostered the concept of private-woman, public-man, women's public
appearances would become an important issue of concern.[1] Women's
public appearances would contribute to the enlargement of their sphere
beyond the domestic realm.

Women's public appearances were often linked to the populist nature
of Methodism and in many ways mirrored John Wesley's reform of
Calvinism through Methodism. Methodism began in England during
the 1730s when John and Charles Wesley attempted to reform Calvinism
by emphasizing their belief in the importance of Christian discipline,
devotion and concern for the poor. Wesley's experiences ministering to
natives and settlers in the Georgian colony in America had convinced
him that through a willingness to believe in God or through faith, any
person would receive "perfect love, entire sanctification or holiness."

The believer would be completely transformed by this change, resulting in a holiness that was practical and social.[2]

Many Methodist women described holiness, or the "warming of the heart," as enabling them to let the regenerating grace of the Holy Spirit take over them. Often this regenerating grace allowed the women to express concern for others outside the household, thus taking precedence over the domestic responsibilities that were the very backbone of Victorian culture. When women acted upon their concerns, it meant that their grace was visible and that they had been touched by the Holy Spirit. The intensity of the "warming of the heart" signaled justification from God that the woman should act upon her holiness in the practical and social manner that Wesley had prescribed. When hearts were warmed, women could interpret this to mean that God was affirming their wish to engage in fund-raising despite social opposition to women in public.[3]

Each time that women missionaries worked in public for the missionary cause, they contributed to stretching the limits of their sphere. Unlike suffragists, who relied upon conservative tactics to compensate for radical goals, churchwomen could lead a more public existence because they were more often perceived as the embodiment of civic virtue. While simultaneously conforming to Victorian gender norms, churchwomen posed a variety of challenges to the idea that the public realm was a male domain.[4]

Piety, or loving obedience and service to God and humanity, was the motivating force behind the activities of nineteenth-century Methodist women involved with missionary work. It was the core impetus for female missionaries in the field who served as educators and medical workers, and those who organized, built and supported female missionary societies at home. These women can best be viewed as a "sisterhood" held together primarily by each member's awareness of a shared belief in the primary importance of serving God and humanity as a priority that might suppress Victorian expectations of a woman's domestic role.

Secular twentieth-century historians have shed light upon how female evangelical missionaries from Baptist, Congregationalist, Methodist and Presbyterian foreign mission groups forestalled improvements in the position of women in American society by their representations of "heathen women." For example, Joan Brumberg's study of late nineteenth-century American evangelical women missionaries of these denominations correlated their depictions of "degraded heathen women," with their assertions of the unique and enviable position of American women. Brumberg postulated that the missionaries' denial of American female restrictions, and the positing of "heathen" women as the "degraded other" had the effect of retarding the implementation of real improvements in the position of women in American society.[5]

Alongside the forces described by Brumberg are seeds of change which would be understood more easily if each denomination of missionary workers would be considered individually. Indeed, Protestant women may be better understood if we cease to view them simply as one coherent group of religious women.[6] Consequently, I will illustrate how many Methodist women's interpretations of piety could not only reinforce traditional notions of women's inferior place but simultaneously pose challenge to male-imposed restrictions.[7]

One can argue that some of their contemporaries should have viewed the Methodist sisterhood as threatening in order for them to have represented a force for challenge to male dominance. Evidence suggests that women active in missionary activities were indeed perceived by some as having ignored their domestic obligations, a serious charge among Victorians. This meant that churchwomen encountered obstacles as they engaged in fund-raising activities for their missionary societies. At an 1884 Methodist Conference in Baltimore, Maryland, one male observer emphasized that a churchwoman should not use her special roles and influence to gain prominence, thus ignoring her special work.[8] In 1889, a minister observed that some women "are so absorbed with "the higher Christian life" that they have no time nor talent for looking after the tidiness of their children, the efficiency and comfort of their husbands. . . ."[9] The Southern Methodist editor and writer Mrs. Sarah Butler noted that the strongest deterrent against the work of women for missions was the "chivalrous feeling that Southern women should retain their old-time unobtrusiveness, without any desire to assert their own personality . . . or engage in anything . . . that would call them out of their sheltered homes."[10]

While this view suggested that some individuals found women's religious work in public threatening, thereby proving that it did challenge societal norms, this threat was not pervasive enough to prevent large numbers of women from becoming interested in the missionary movement and the public work related to it. In fact, it was because Victorian society largely perceived female piety as conservative that the women's religious efforts can be seen as having planted seeds of empowerment among the sisters. Moreover, I believe that the sisters' subtle challenges to Victorian separate sphere dictates were made possible by their conservative garb as churchwomen.[11]

The societal perception of churchwomen's conservative nature stemmed from the belief that a woman's primary role was that of Christian mother, the inculcator and protector of correct Protestant values among family members. An extension of this domestic expression of piety was the notion that a religious woman's primary responsibility, either as a missionary or as a supporter, was to help evangelize "heathen" women. As mothers, these women in foreign lands were also conservators of religion who could potentially keep Protestantism alive worldwide.[12]

Protestant women at home were seen as fulfilling their mandate to Christian motherhood by supporting the missionary cause with both their monies and labors. Victorian society perceived a compatibility between a woman's religiosity, the spreading of both domestic and international Protestantism, and the belief that Protestant women, identified primarily by their role as mothers, were to remain in the private sphere.

While churchwomen were predominantly perceived as conservative, their missionary work was also an impetus for a number of endeavors which, in aggregate, attacked the most critical foundations of Victorian female identity. As such, what I call "empowerment-through-piety" can be viewed as a subtle vehicle for women's traversal from the private to the public world.

While the exact number of societies established is not completely known,[13] religious women's challenges to private sphere restrictions began in the 1810s and were connected with their efforts to organize, hold meetings and raise funds for missionary work.[14] Eventually the women would create a number of benevolent societies, local and state temperance organizations and missionary societies. The rise of women's missionary societies was often a response to the existing work of male Methodists, but the implementation of women's goals often countered the premise of male authority in the public realm.

In 1819 Mary Mason founded the New York Female Missionary Society, auxiliary to the male Methodist Missionary and Bible Society which had been established the same year.[15] Mason described herself as having spent her young adulthood rebelling against her parents' wish that she take an interest in parties, rather than books and benevolence. She found the impetus for rebellion after having a conversion experience, which prompted her to go from house to house, spreading the gospel. Mason noted that her behavior would have "carried her to the stake" in earlier decades.[16]

As directress, Mason appealed to churchwomen to do their utmost for the Lord, and their missionary society, leaving "nothing unattempted which promises to promote the advancement of the Redeemer's Kingdom." In order to support missionary activities among Indian tribes in the United States and Canada, and eventually missionary work in Africa, the women of Mason's Society engaged, not only in such traditional tasks as spinning and sewing, but also in door to door fund-raising, considered unwomanly behavior.[17]

News of the New York Society's work prompted women in Baltimore, Boston, Philadelphia and several cities in New York State to emulate their fellow churchwomen and establish their own auxiliaries to the existing male Methodist Missionary and Bible Society. In aggregate, the women's fund-raising efforts would provide over twenty-thousand dollars to the Methodist Episcopal Board during the first half-century of its existence.[18]

The women's Liberia Missionary Society was created in response to the Methodist Episcopal Board's first missionary appointment to Africa. Organized in 1840, with Mrs. S. B. Fox as its president, the women of the Society went from house to house to raise money for the missionary cause, however, according to an 1881 account by Methodist author Mary Sparkes Wheeler, they were "often persecuted and rejected." They persevered despite this opposition because, as Wheeler noted, "they met for deliberation and prayer" and eventually "the divine power over-shadowed them."

> Their hearts were strangely warmed—a baptism of love and power fell upon them—and taking this as an evidence of divine approval, they set out with much enthusiasm to collect what they could for the enterprise.[19]

This "baptism of love and power" enabled the women to continue their work when they encountered opposition. As Mrs. Fox explained, the "blessing of God" had resulted in an increased prosperity which eventually prompted the "prejudice to give way," allowing the women to continue their work.[20]

The Ladies' China Missionary Society, established in response to the Methodist Episcopal Board's initiation of work in China in 1848, likewise pointed to the regenerating grace of the Holy Spirit as that which gave them the power to counter the protestations of churchmen. Inspired by what the society's founder identified as a lack of "avenue for woman's work in the Methodist Episcopal Church," the women were reported to have worked diligently in the face of adversity. One observer of the society in its early stages noted that the women were a "feeble band," yet in another sense they were "strong" due to their faith and determination. According to Mary Sparkes Wheeler, faith gave women power as they "struggled on through opposition and difficulties."[21]

Much opposition stemmed from churchmen who believed that an independent woman's organization was an infringement, not only on Church usage, but the absolute rights of the missionary board. Despite this response, the ladies were neither dissuaded nor disloyal, and they attained a degree of influence. The new society raised three-hundred dollars per year for ten years for the Methodist Episcopal board. By 1859 they would contribute to the establishment of a girls' school in Foochow, in the Chinese province of Fukien, and they would even see to it that two single women missionary sisters from New Jersey, Sarah and Beulah Woolston, be sent to administer the school.[22]

The Woolston sisters had been educated at Wesleyan Female College in Wilmington, Delaware, an institution which had inspired female missionary interest beginning in the early nineteenth century. In 1846, graduates of the college delivered an address to their Alumnae Association and the result was a reorganization of that group into a Woman's Foreign Missionary Society that would inspire student interest in missions. Wheeler described the members of the society as talented speakers, skillful in their deliberations.[23]

Wheeler's description of these female society members' oratorical endeavors is at odds with Victorian America's emphasis upon a woman's social relatedness and the expectation that she work for the good of her society rather than herself. While oratory was considered an individual achievement and most women dared not speak in public, piety allowed some women to circumvent this constraint.[24]

Their Southern sisters paralleled the efforts of the northern women in these public endeavors, which often involved public speaking.[25] Little is known of the first Southern Methodist female effort at missionary work that began in 1824 when a home missionary society was organized in Jonesboro, Tennessee; however, women who established missionary societies during the 1830s were chronicled in female Methodist missionary histories.

Methodist editor and writer, Sarah Butler, noted in 1904 that the women of the Female Missionary Society of Lynchburg, Virginia were zealous and skillful managers and speakers: Their annual reports were eloquent and powerful. They were excellent fund-raisers: collections were taken at annual meetings, and receipts were reported to be considerable. For example, a total of $579.10 was raised by 1839.[26] Expansion of women's roles during the Civil War prompted a postwar proliferation of women's missionary societies.

One southern lady's commentary regarding wartime changes, a classic among female Methodists, reflected the women's awareness of the importance of oratory and its capacity to broaden a woman's sphere of activity. Mrs. E. C. Dowdell wrote to Bishop James O. Andrew in 1861, taking note of how patriotism had inspired female relief work "made necessary by the battles fought on Southern soil." Dowdell remarked upon how this work affected society's view of women: they could "preside over large assemblies, read compositions" and present flags to "plaudits" of congratulations. Dowdell observed what contemporary historians have reiterated: during the Civil War women were allowed to challenge the notion that political consciousness and an identification with the fate of the nation were exclusively male preserves.[27] She believed there was a lesson to be learned.

Dowdell suggested that churchwomen emulate the behavior of patriotic females and make themselves just as "conspicuous." As if prophetically predicting that postbellum women would later be deprived of the patrioticly motivated surplus energy outlet that they had enjoyed during the war years, Dowdell urged preventative action. She insisted that a Woman's Missionary Society be created, reasoning that if women were allowed to appear in public for their country then they might also do so for the "cause" of God; and if society accepted a more public role for women justified by patriotism, then it should accept one motivated by piety.[28]

Dowdell's observation is important when considered in conjunction with the knowledge that Methodist women were already organizing at the local level prior to the Civil War. It suggests that women's work during that war simply accelerated already existing trends for female organization.[29]

The proliferation of female missionary societies in the post-Civil War era was also precipitated by the increasing level of religious energy possessed by women in the decades surrounding the Civil War. Historians have described this religious energy but have not explored its connection to the proliferation of female missionary societies and the public speaking opportunities it could often afford women. As historian Timothy Smith has shown, women were active participants in the religious revivals, Holiness Movement and camp meetings of the 1850s and 1860s.[30]

Camp meetings took place when hundreds of men and women would gather at a clearing, set up tents and attend revivals for a few days. While these meetings were particularly suited to frontier areas, they were not only confined there. One can view them as having taken place in what contemporary historians would define as a public arena. Hence, camp meetings allowed women equal access to, what was by middle-class Victorian standards, a male-designated domain.

While itinerant preachers were the main focus of attention at camp meetings, the gatherings were most distinctive for the uninhibitedness they provoked among participants. Nathan Hatch described one account of the role of ministers and the audience reaction:

> to have the power of God "strike fire" over a mass audience; they encouraged uncensored testimonials by persons without respect to age, gender or race . . .

the public sharing of private ecstasy . . . overt physical display and emotional release . . .[31]

Camp meeting testimonials were likewise at odds with Victorian America's emphasis upon Victorian constraints against female public speaking. At camp meetings, women found a public voice and sense of individuality. A woman's heart-felt piety could find expression through her public speaking at a revival. This may have been especially true for women Methodists, with their denomination's strong laical tradition, or emphasis upon the importance of the layperson.[32] For example, Nancy Cott's study of New England revivals found that while from 1780–1835, Methodists encouraged women to pray aloud in public, ministers of other denominations strengthened restrictions against this practice.[33]

On the other hand, some evidence suggests that the women's experiences at camp meetings during the postbellum period were neither confined to the Methodists nor without earlier precedents. Historian Virginia Brereton has noted that as early as 1803, women found the public conversion experience an impetus for greater "self-confidence" and "inner-strength." One female convert reported:

> I had the strength of God to talk to them; my tongue seemed to be let loose and my heart was enlarged; it seemed that my mouth was filled with arguments; the scriptures flowed into my mind, text after text. . . . It being in the city, two hundred had collected before I had done speaking.[34]

Historian Nathan Hatch described a young female New Hampshire schoolteacher who, after a conversion inspired by another woman in 1818, traveled 15,000 miles within a decade, encountered "a score of women preachers among Christians, Freewill Baptists, Universalists, and Methodists and called for more female laborers in the Gospel harvestfield."[35]

The activities of the women who helped to establish the post-Civil War Northern and Southern Women's Foreign Missionary societies may be understood in light of this background of "religious pluralism" which afforded women an opportunity for self-expression. Their activities reflected the ways in which pious convictions could triumph when pitted against women's consciousness of the conflicting Victorian taboo against oratory and its suggestion of a more public role for women.

The "intrepid eight" who organized the Northern Woman's Foreign Missionary Society of the Methodist Episcopal Church in March of 1869 were the wives of bishops, representative of the middle-class woman of Victorian America.[36] However, the tenuous relationship between the women's "public" duties and their relegation to "private" restrictions, came to be significantly altered with their increased role in the societies and subsequent participation in the camp meetings of the 1860s and 1870s.

Mrs. Clementina Butler accompanied her husband, a missionary for the Methodist Episcopal Church, to India in 1856 and helped establish a mission, which would have 17 missionary members and 117 church members by 1864. That year Butler returned home to suggest to the well-to-do Methodist women of her Tremont Street Church that they should concern themselves with women of foreign lands. While the women initially preferred to continue their work with Boston's poor, Butler employed several means of persuasion, eventually winning over the Tremont Street churchwomen.

Evincing an ethnocentrism that was common among missionaries, Mrs. Butler and her husband spoke to the group about the burdens faced by Hindu and Muslim women. She spoke highly of the female missionary society created by Congregationalists in 1868 and showed the Tremont Street women the Constitution of the Congregational Woman's Board of Missions, a copy of their magazine, *Life and Light*, and a leaflet on Congregationalist women's zenana work. By 1869 Butler organized the Woman's Foreign Missionary Society of the Methodist Episcopal Church.[37]

Many male church members, including the corresponding secretary of the General Missionary Society, Dr. John Durbin, were opposed to the organization of a woman's society. These churchmen believed that the fragmentation of fund-raising efforts would provide unwelcome competition to the Methodist Episcopal Board. Negotiations between the new women's society and the board resulted in an agreement published by the Women's Foreign Missionary Society's first issue of its publication: *The Heathen Woman's Friend*, in June of 1869. This agreement stipulated that the General Society would review all appropriations and appointments and that funds not be raised by collections or subscriptions taken during any church services or in any "promiscuous," public meeting, where the audience was composed of both men and women. Rather, funds should be raised by "securing Members, Life Members, Honorary Managers, and Patrons" in such a way as "would not interfere with the Parent Society."[38]

While the women agreed to seek churchmen's approval for their work, significant evidence exists that, rather than passively confining themselves to a restricted sphere, the Women's Foreign Missionary Society (hereafter WFMS) cleverly subverted the Methodist Episcopal Board's attempts at control. For example, after a year of receiving monies from Massachusetts women and forming auxiliaries, the WFMS had its first meeting to discuss the appointment of its first missionary, Isabella Thoburn. At this 1870 meeting, Mrs. Butler expressed her strong argument that a medical missionary should accompany Miss Thoburn. Some WFMS ladies objected, fearful that insufficient monies might impede the departure of both educational missionary Miss Isabella Thoburn and a medical missionary. When these women "counseled prudence," one WFMS lady rose to give a speech regarded as "historic" by Methodist women. In a language, which clearly evinced her view of women's public place and reluctant deference to nineteenth-century female dictates of consumption and feminity, she argued:[39]

> Shall we lose Miss Thoburn because we have not the needed money in our hands to send her? No! Rather let us walk the streets of Boston in calico dresses, if need be, and save the expense of more costly apparel.[40]

For married ladies in 1870s Victorian America, support for a woman's avowal to walk the streets were not commonplace, signaling their changing views concerning the significance of the word "public." Moreover, their determination to wear calico rather than the more costly apparel, reflected their willingness to present themselves outside of societal parameters of feminine acceptability.

According to historian Mary Ryan, beginning in the 1870s, the participation of women in public was marked by an emphasis upon the creation of a spectacle of femininity. An observer at the 1883 celebration of the opening of the Brooklyn Bridge noted "the sartorial splendor of the ladies, their pale, frothy garments and their fluttering handkerchiefs presenting a veritable phalanx of white." Mostly seen in attire evoking goddess images, women were more commonly seen carrying flowers, their presence symbolizing passivity.[41] The WFMS ladies' willingness to forego the more "costly" attire can be taken as an act of rebellion against the passive image and elite class more commonly associated with postbellum women's public appearances.

The woman's avowal to wear "calico" represented her rejection of female dictates of pious consumption. Women were disregarding the more costly, socially sanctioned apparel for calico, a cheap cotton worn in "heathen" lands, the foreign fields of China and India. As early as the late eighteenth century, Protestant preachers had asserted that beauty, and later materialism, or the accumulation of luxury goods, including clothing, was civilizing, socializing and conducive to the awakening of higher sentiments. By the third decade of the nineteenth century, consumer refinement and gracious materiality had become a specifically feminine province, the sign of feminine influence and presence, and a sign of male respect for feminine sensibility among middle class Victorians.[42] The ladies' willingness to appear in calico indicated an abandonment of the female refinement the women knew to be expected by middle-class Victorian males.

Viewed in a broader context, the WFMS ladies' breach of etiquette suggests their activities had already, by 1870, broadened their understanding of the word "public." This changing conception reflects the increasingly public activities of the women.

The structure of the WFMS had much to do with its increasingly broad base and far-reaching proliferation. The plan for this structure had grown out of regional rivalries. The New York women who had raised money to send Clara Swain to India were fearful that their society would become subservient to the Boston society. The New York women elicited an agreement with the Methodist Parent Board stipulating that each woman's foreign missionary society branch established would have representation in one central authoritative body, an Executive Committee made up of representatives of all branches.[43]

Eliminating the potential for power struggle among branches, the WFMS saw increasing growth. After the first year, the societies proliferated to such an extent that more than half came from Western states such as Indiana, Ilinois, Michigan and Wisconsin.[44]

During the first decade of the Northern female society's existence, the organizing for the missionary cause went on at camp meetings in such diverse locations as Martha's Vineyard, Massachusetts; Albion, Michigan; Round Lake, New York; Clifton Springs, New York; Ocean Grove, New Jersey; Lakeside, Ohio; Lancaster, Ohio; Tippecanoe Battle Ground, Indiana; Lake Bluff, Illinois and Silver Lake, Michigan, recognized by religious historians as Methodist/Holiness watering holes. The rhetoric at these camp meetings was so persuasive as to encourage many women to join missionary organizations.[45]

Biographies of women Methodist leaders often note that their subject's inspiration originated at a camp meeting. For example, one missionary society founder described herself as having found inspiration at the age of sixteen years old when she "embraced religion in East Tennessee at Muddy Creek Camp Ground."[46] The experience of missionary wife and WFMS founder Mrs. Clementina Butler at one camp meeting sheds light upon why a female audience could find such an event appealing. Butler, who traveled and organized auxiliary Methodist societies throughout New York, made her first appearance as a public speaker at an 1869 camp meeting in Sing Sing, New York. The men had just terminated their meeting, and were prompted to allow a meeting "for women only." Mrs. Butler spoke successfully, charming everyone with her "Irish wit," then raised a collection. Butler's initial rebellion, raising a collection, was enabled by her adherence to the Parent Board's rule that females not address "promiscuous" gatherings. She adhered to this rule by subverting male power. There had been a half-dozen "curious" men in the audience, but Butler had had them ejected by a policeman. Having ordered the physical removal of a group of males from their designated realm of "public" dominion, Mrs. Butler was able to create a "non-promiscuous assembly" of women only in keeping with the WFMS's agreement with the Parent Board. In the process she had caused quite a stir.

When her husband, Dr. William Butler, arrived, concerned about his wife's safety in all the commotion, he attempted to enter the meeting area but found that he too was barred from entering.[47] Later, when Dr. Durbin, of the Methodist Episcopal Board, complained that contrary to agreement, a "public collection" had been held, Mrs. Butler objected: "a meeting from which men were excluded could not be called public." What would become a legendary account among Methodist women was Butler's reaction to Dr. Durbin's reproach. She noted that she took a "wigging" for "holding public meetings and taking up public collections." Durbin insisted that he "heard at every turn that the ladies had been holding great meetings at Sing Sing Camp Meeting and collecting large sums of money." Butler recalled that he "was in a great fuss," but rather than express concern, she "laughed at him," adding: "I am ready to do it again!"[48]

Butler provided "much publicity" for the "society in the camp meetings then in vogue" by jousting a few curious men and excluding even her own husband from the male dominated "public" sphere of influence.[49] She had not only managed to shift the boundaries established by males by asserting female authority, but had done so by speaking without any of the embarassment or self-deprecation that historians attribute to "self-denying" Victorian women.

By the 1870s when secular women did speak to audiences without embarassment, their decorum and messages were placid ones, a tribute to the males who happened to be present. According to Mary Ryan, the women "posed behind a feminized facade." For example, one woman "delivered a pretty little address" as she presented a banner to the Benevolent Sons of Louisiana in 1871. Ryan explains that this comportment was necessary because women's "forays into public space during the nineteenth century" subjected them "to intense male scrutiny."[50]

As a pious woman, Butler could provide a contrast to the secular, patriotic and feminine work of late nineteenth-century women in public. The female audience who had had the pleasure of viewing Mrs. Butler's performance was treated to an example of female subversion of male power, albeit condoned by pious motivation. That the episode provided publicity for the society illustrates how WFMS workers, acting through piety, were able to broaden the parameters of the word "public" to women audience members and those who would read about the meeting.

Butler's confidence in female oratory is further illustrated by her encounter with the Methodist Frances E. Willard. When the young Willard was asked to speak on behalf of the WFMS in the early 1870s, Butler observed the young woman's "natural" discomfort. In response, she immediately set out with gentle persuasion and helped Willard discover "she had a voice and could give a message." Willard went on to establish the Women's Christian Temperance Union and become an avid worker for the cause of woman's suffrage.[51]

Butler's belief is representative of the sisterhood's emphasis: piety took precedence over Victorian reservedness. The need to raise monies for the missionary cause required that women set aside their inhibitions and enter a designated male realm.

Southern Methodist women introduced conceptions of a woman's right to speak and organize for missionary work with as much force as their Northern sisters. Like the married women founders of the WFMS, missionary society leaders in Nashville, Tennessee, and Baltimore, Maryland, were inspired by the activities of women speakers in Northern areas and from different denominations.

The initial goal of Mrs. Margaret Kelley and Mrs. Willie Elizabeth McGavock, two well-known Southern Methodist missionary leaders, was to forge ties among the small, scattered missionary societies that had formed in the early to mid-1800s and continued to exist in the postbellum South. McGavock noted that her inspiration came not only from Margaret Kelley's fund-raising activities and efforts dating back to 1858, but also from Congregationalist women who gave powerful public speeches for the cause of "heathen" women. For example, in 1875, as Corresponding Secretary of the Nashville society, McGavock described attending a large meeting of the Woman's Missionary Society of the Congregational Church in Chicago. There were 1500 in the audience and she recalled that there was "not even standing room" in the aisles. McGavock was impressed that it was a woman who presided over this "vast throng," of women and that from 9:00 A.M. to 1:00 P.M. "many women missionaries from different parts of the world" made captivating addresses "by their eloquence, their earnestness, and the simple recital of their experiences and labor. . . ." She noted that the addresses were "not written but spoken with womanly modesty and dignity." McGavock told her Methodist sisters that if they "could have seen the effect on that listening multitude, [their] hearts would have been fired with fresh zeal," as hers had been. Observing the scene, McGavock asked: "Why cannot our Southern women, so brave and true in the ordinary affairs of life, thus organize, and by united effort make themselves felt as a power for Christ in the land?"[52]

In 1876, when Mrs. McGavock began to petition church members in an effort to prepare for the Southern Methodist General Conference of 1878, her objective was to attain recognition for the establishment of a large Woman's Missionary Society and to raise money to pay for the expenses of a woman missionary to China for one year. The correspondence resulting from McGavock's appeals demonstrates how women's missionary literature could suggest a change in male conceptions of women and women's conceptions of themselves. One bishop sent a $125 check to Mrs. McGavock, explaining in a note that his wife had "made a public presentation of the cause, reading your [McGavock's] letter and making brief addresses, a novelty which attracted more attention and elicited more interest than an address from me or any of the pastors."[53]

Another churchman wrote to McGavock of his realization that "it is a mistake not to give woman's work in missions prominence; and if this is 'woman's rights,' I am prepared to give her the fullest liberty. Those who oppose it ought to get out from under the wheels of this chariot, for it will not stop!"[54]

Mrs. McGavock noted the extent of female interest in public evangelical work:

> The Methodist Episcopal Church, South, seems to be waking up to the fact that women are both able and willing to render effective service in evangelizing the world. Almost every week letters come from women in different States, asking for information in reference to organizing societies.[55]

Immediately after the action of the General Conference to organize a Woman's Missionary Society on 23 May 1878, McGavock, named the corresponding secretary, wrote to everyone whose address she could obtain, and "packages of missionary literature were sent by hundreds and thousands," showing what united women had done for the evangelization of the world thus far. The new president, Juliana Hayes, was eager to travel and organize new societies.[56]

Southern women like Mrs. Dowdell viewed the work of Hayes and others like her as important for swaying those people who had read, or heard quoted portions of St. Paul's writings about women "learning in silence" and "usurping authority." These proponents of a more active woman's public role, sought to educate those who had "never read or heard of those women that labored . . . in the gospel."[57] Mrs. Dowdell's admiration for Juliana Hayes had inspired her 1861 letter to Bishop Andrews.

Southern editor Mrs. Sarah Butler described Juliana Hayes as having been "ubiquitous" during the early "organizing" years of the Southern WFMS. Hayes was "credited with having attended the organizational meetings in eleven different conferences" and "generating enthusiasm for the cause wherever she went." Butler noted that she was perceived as "intellectual," and intelligent, with a "never-failing readiness of speech" bolstered by a "quick wit and graceful habit of repartee in meeting objections." A vivacious woman, whose talks were irresistible to audiences, Juliana Hayes was no demure Southern lady or modest Victorian: rather, she had a "keen, humorous reply in argument."[58]

In 1878, the sixty-five year old Hayes traveled from Maryland to Texas, speaking to thousands of audiences of women and men, and collecting large sums of money. Her memoirs recalled one series of four-day meetings: "I spoke three times on Sunday. The Holy Spirit seemed to own my efforts. Fixed attention characterized the congregations. I have organized three auxiliaries."[59]

A classic female Methodist account of Hayes is one man's reaction at a Florida Conference:

> the gentleman who had been asked to introduce her refused because he thought women should be seen and not heard in public. But he was so moved by her address that he changed his opinion and became a strong advocate of women and their work.[60]

Southern female missionary leader Alice Culler Cobb would become a salaried secretary for the Woman's Board in the early twentieth century. She too is an example of the type of Southern woman who inspired support for women's more public role through organization for the missionary cause. In 1879, Cobb was President of the Conference Missionary Society of Perry, Georgia, an organization whose aim it was to link up the scattered Southern female Methodist auxiliaries with each other and with the year old Woman's Board based in Nashville.

In her capacity as associate secretary of the Southern WFMS, Cobb held meetings and gave talks to raise money for a girls' school in China. Significantly, Cobb's 1925 biography, by her niece, Mary Culler White, emphasized her frequent public speaking engagements, yet sought to distinguish her style from that of feminists. White noted that Cobb spoke without the characteristic presentation of a "well-known woman's organization whose public speakers were in her estimation loud of voice, and masculine in manner." This obvious allusion to feminists meant that White felt the need to protect her aunt against charges that she was unwomanly. According to White, Cobb's speeches were delivered with "clearness and force" and through this representation as a strong woman, White felt that Cobb could encourage timid women to speak and assume leadership positions. Cobb tried not to appear too radical or threatening to scare women away; rather, as White noted, Cobb was careful to speak in the "low voice of the typical southern woman."[61]

Mary Culler White's appreciation for her aunt's speaking abilities appeared related to her own recollections of meeting another woman missionary leader, Belle Bennett, president of the Woman's Home Mission Society and leader for Southern women's laity rights. At an annual meeting of the Woman's missionary conference of South Georgia, during the first decade of this century, Belle Bennett encouraged White to speak. Unable to forget her pride at the personal interest Bennett had shown in her, White credited that experience as both having given her an increased sense of self-worth and the impetus to become a foreign missionary to China.[62]

Missionary society activities and meetings not only encouraged women to speak but also allowed women in both the Northern and Southern WFMS auxiliaries access to a broader range of information not normally accessible in Victorian American. As a result, what this study terms cultivation-through-piety, suggested to women that they could influence, the larger world outside the household. Northern and Southern Methodist society women introduced the idea that piety justified a female education for purposes outside the parameters of household tasks.

Women workers for the missionary cause expressed the view that piety required female cultivation. Women should improve themselves and other women by the thorough development of their mental faculties so that they might more fully serve God and humanity. While the women expressed an emphasis upon service as their primary motivation, their philosophies toward women's education were in direct contravention to the Victorian precept that all women's activities should be directed toward strengthening domestic abilities.

Exponents of the female cultivation-through-piety ideal offered alternatives which differed from those philosophies considered acceptable to most people in Victorian America. By the postbellum period, many people were in agreement that women should be educated, but few concurred with the idea that this instruction should prepare them for anything but domestic or practical duties. The ideal of "True Womanhood" emphasized that women's education should prepare them for a domestic role.[63] On the other hand, the competing ideal of "Real Womanhood" emphasized the need for a practical education, enabling the female student to eventually earn a living under optimal conditions.[64] The cultivation-through-piety ideal offered a third option, not yet considered by secular scholars of woman's history.

As early as 1870, one year after the publication of the WFMS's magazine, *The Heathen Woman's Friend*, Mrs. Jennie Fowler Willing, a corresponding secretary for a western branch of the WFMS, complained that there was not enough appealing literature on missions. It was not enough to have statistics illustrating the number of conversions on the foreign field. Willing suggested that society members read missionary periodicals and books written by those women who were experts in the field. She urged women to establish "missionary reading circles in every auxiliary society," and prepare papers in order to discuss this material. "When I first invited the ladies to write and read," Willing noted, "they thought me wild!"[65]

One important result of Willing's idea for a more challenging arena for women missionary society members was "Uniform Readings," which came as a supplement to the *Heathen Woman's Friend*. With "Uniform Study," female Methodist auxiliary members were provided with three months of instruction on the history and general characteristics of the country and people in each foreign field, then that nation's general missionary history, and thirdly, the facts regarding its Methodist Episcopal Missions. According to WFMS leaders, the use of encyclopedias, "histories and magazine articles" provided auxiliary members with "a liberal education."[66] Since the *Heathen Woman's Friend* was a well-circulated publication, with subscriptions expanding from 3,500 in 1869 to 21,000 in 1870, and 92,591 by 1929, this "liberal education" proliferated significantly among society members.[67]

Asked by their societies to serve the world, female auxiliary members had first to increase their knowledge of it. Time spent learning about the world was time *not* spent enhancing female domestic skills. The educational itinerary was an appealing one to women eager to broaden their horizons. In an 1873 issue of *Heathen Woman's Friend*, one female Methodist explained that "we must have something to talk about better than cake-making or flounces."[68]

The women's opportunities for critical thinking and for speaking publicly within their auxiliaries served to broaden their personal sense of influence to an area usually perceived as male-dominated. The auxiliary members were urged to think about peoples and situations outside of the context of the household, and encouraged to study mission fields in ways that did more than just exercise "their mental muscles."[69]

Alluding to the spiritual liberation afforded women at Methodist "love feasts," female readers of an 1879 issue of *Heathen Woman's Friend* were encouraged to approach their monthly meetings, no longer as a "love feast" but as a "thought feast." They were urged to think of those people in far-off countries as "neighbors" whose "circumstances, conditions, civilizations" needed to be understood.[70]

Southern Methodist missionary auxiliary leaders' pedagogical techniques matched those of their northern sisters. Southern female leaders sought to provide women with factual information, as well as lessons on how to organize and direct the movement. Revealing her motivations, Mrs. McGavock complained in 1877 that while the women were "able and willing to render effective service in evangelizing the world," they were also "waiting for the other to lead."[71] McGavock viewed education as a means for providing churchwomen with a sense that they could take the initiative rather than simply wait passively for outside direction.

The provision for "reading circles" and the communication of "intelligence" concerning the foreign field was made in the first Southern Women's missionary society auxiliary constitution of 1878. Sarah Butler, the biographer of Mrs. Juliana Hayes and Mrs. D. H. McGavock and chronicler of the *History of the Woman's Foreign Missionary Society*, was editor of an important periodical, the *Woman's Missionary Advocate*, which constituted a major source for auxiliary members' knowledge of the foreign field. Home field supporters also learned through religious leaflets, textbooks written by missionaries and articles in the *Christian Advocate*, an important source for the views of Methodist missionaries in the United States.[72]

Like the *Heathen Woman's Friend* and the *Woman's Missionary Friend*, the *Woman's Missionary Advocate*'s circulation grew significantly. From its inception in 1880, to its termination in 1910, subscribers grew from 6,000 to 22,000.[73] After 1883, requests for the leaflets and pamphlets published by the Literature Department of the Southern WFMS had far exceeded the 35,000 produced since 1881. This demand did not diminish with time. By 1896, 20,000 of each monthly leaflet and pamphlet were being issued and editors found it increasingly difficult to produce sufficient copies.[74]

Why did women missionary supporters find the educational material appealing? While the readings furthered Southern home field supporters' knowledge of foreign lands, challenging the patriarchal order of white men over white women, as Joan Brumberg has shown, it did so by simultaneously positing "third world women" as the antithetical "Other."[75] Thus, the effect of the reading material was to both challenge and sustain Victorian middle-class conceptions of order.

While the viewpoints of readers are difficult to determine, women leaders' educational ideals were clearly reflected in the material. Laura

Askew Haygood, missionary educator, administrator and 1891 founder of the McTyeire School of Shanghai, published her views of women's education in society in 1884, prior to her departure for China. Haygood believed that women had a large role in the public world and that household demands should not be the center of a woman's being. She urged that "no course of study can be too advanced, no learning too deep, no culture too broad, to help in the making of the perfect woman," who would be "moved to compassion" for the world.[76]

Alice Culler Cobb's 1863 salutation address at Georgia Wesleyan Female College asserted that the assumption of radical difference among genders had already been refuted: "woman has been gradually brought to a knowledge of the revealed truths of science, and elevated to the high position which she now occupies in society." Cobb declared the death of the old view that "hapless female was supposed to be well freighted for time's hazardous voyage if she possessed a knowledge of the lower branches of an English education, could finger well upon a stringed instrument." That view had been replaced by recognition that "woman is no longer denied her right and title to the thorough cultivation and development of her intellectual faculties."[77]

The combination of activities meant to cultivate knowledge of world history through reading, writing and speaking would be neither in keeping with the ideals of "True Womanhood" or "Real Womanhood." They would be neither practical for earning a living nor beneficial to a woman in the household. The activities would allow women to experience and initiate occupation of the public sphere, to develop a self-confidence mirroring that possessed by professional women and to articulate thoughts regarding the wider world outside the household—a world that was largely occupied by men.[78]

Undoubtedly, the educational efforts of female Methodists within the auxiliaries fulfilled American churchwomen's need for conversation outside of the parameters of baking and keeping house. While we cannot know with certainly exactly how women supporters interpreted the empowerment-through-piety ideal, it is important to understand that it was an aspect of the message they received through the representation, and at times, direct expressions of leaders in the missionary movement.

Women Methodists belonged to the largest Protestant denomination in the United States during the nineteenth century. In addition, they also constituted the most significant segment of what collectively was the most sizable female communications network in existence during that time. Interdenominationally, Women's missionary societies were the largest of any group of woman's movements by the late nineteenth century.[79] How widespread and numerous female were the home field supporters of women like Ailie Gale?

By 1896, after nearly twenty-five years, it was estimated that the total number of women belonging to all of the foreign missionary societies was close to 600,000. In comparison, by 1890 the National American Woman Suffrage Association (NAWSA) had numbered only 7,000 members, while the Woman's Christian Temperance Union (WCTU) would number only 168,000 by 1899. By 1915 female membership in foreign missionary societies would rise to over three million and the Methodists would become the largest subset of this group, both in numbers and in church members recruited.[80]

The Methodist society's growth had been impressive, with over 150,000 members by 1895, 267,000 in 1910 (at a time when the NAWSA's membership was only 75,000) and over 500,000 by 1920. In 1913, at a time when the church itself was the predominant organization in which most early-twentieth-century women were involved, one of every eight churchwomen belonged to the WFMS.[81]

Methodist women had often spoken of the necessity of obtaining small mites from their numerous supporters, perceiving this as proof that all women's hearts would be touched by the cause. In Mrs. McGavock's 1893 address to the Southern women's board's annual session, for example, she reminded them that the society's income came not "from the abundance of the rich, but largely from the penuries of the poor," and that there was never a gift which amounted to as much as $5,000.[82] As Ailie Gale would understand several decades later, McGavock knew that these small sums insured the popularity of the movement. Moreover, the small sums involved did not preclude women from making a formidable financial contribution to the foreign missionary effort, enough to eventually allow women a measure of freedom from the dominance of their parent board.

From its creation in 1878, to the death in 1895 of Mrs. McGavock, the Southern WFMS grew to 70,000 members, supporting 38 foreign missionaries, 109 teachers and helpers, 11 Bible women, twelve boarding schools, and one hospital. The total raised by the Southern WFMS until 1895 was $853,024.68.[83]

The Northern Methodists, the largest of the women's societies, outdid all other female missionary organizations, with member contributions totaling nearly one million dollars a year by 1909.[84] By 1912, 35 percent of the total receipts, or $840,000, for the foreign missions of the Methodist Episcopal Church derived from the contributions of the WFMS, whose yearly giving averaged $3.53 per member. In comparison, the contributions of most female societies averaged 20 percent of their respective Parent Boards' total receipts.[85]

The monies raised were reflective of the popularity of the missionary movement, and especially the Methodist society, for American women. The successes of both the Northern and Southern female societies had important ramifications with regard to relations with the Methodist Episcopal Board. Because the Parent Board could not keep up with all the monies contributed by the female societies, beginning within the first year of its existence in 1869, Methodist women were granted an unrivaled autonomy for the allocation and disbursal of funds.[86] The women of the Northern WFMS would remain autonomous until the 1939 unification of the male and female boards of the Northern and Southern Methodist Episcopal Churches, and the Methodist Protestant Church.

In the Southern Female Society, autonomy was lost in 1910 when the Southern Methodist Episcopal Church General Conference "reorganized all women's mission work under one general board on which women would be given one-third representation."[87] However, the eventual loss of autonomy should not obscure the fact that women's most important victory was the increasing feminization of the missionary movement itself.[88] This feminization is important for historians' understanding of the American public's perceived friendship for China. As the largest portion of missionary supporters and approximately half of the American public, women's attitudes toward China were a force to be reckoned with.

By 1939, when the sentimental attachment of Americans to the Chinese was particularly strong, the Woman's Methodist Missionary Council raised a higher sum for the China Rehabilitation Campaign than did all the Methodist churches combined.[89] This is not surprising, considering the amounts of money raised during the early decades of the century. Through most of the period from 1913 until 1939, the WFMS raised more money for China than did the Methodist Episcopal Board of Missions. In 1912, for example, the WFMS raised $188,141 and the Methodist Episcopal Board raised $153,903. In 1913, the figures were $225,575 and $164,819, respectively.[90]

The amounts raised by the WFMS were especially large, considering these represented an aggregate of small sums donated by the formidable numbers of Methodist women supporters. During the 1920s, at a time when Chinese Nationalism turned virulently anti-Christian, the sums were especially high. In 1922, the WFMS raised $605,855, and the totals for 1923 and 1924, in aggregate, were over $1,000,000. From 1925 to 1932, despite the onset of the depression, the WFMS raised over $400,000 per year. It was not until the depression was well underway in 1934 that yearly appropriations dropped to a little over $300,000 per year, leveling off to $268,020 and $254,182, in 1938 and 1939.[91]

Just as married and single women leaders raised money for the establishment of auxiliaries and the implementation of missionary projects by appealing to supporters as part of a sisterhood, women missionaries like Ailie Gale procured funds for China by addressing shared conceptions of piety. Empowerment-through-piety occurred when the typically womanly endeavor of "social concern," considered an innately female proclivity by many middle-class Victorians, became an unconscious or conscious vehicle for countering patriarchal authority, enabling women to use the tools of the public sphere, fund-raising, speaking and public appearances for piety. Because their motivation for "social concern" was triggered by a discourse relegating non-Western women to an antithetical other, empowerment-through-piety can not be interpreted as a uniform challenge to hierarchical order. Indeed, gender and race are, as Chandra Mohanty has noted "relational terms," and nineteenth-century Methodist women's consciousness of their gender must be seen alongside their depictions of the inferiority of "heathen" women.[92] On the other hand, heeding anthropologist Michele Rosaldo's observation that "woman's place in human social life" should be perceived as the product of the "meaning her activities acquire through concrete social interactions," allows scholars to understand that intertwined with the conservative message of the sisters was a force for change. Hence, Methodist women's proclivity for "social concern" should be understood from the perspective of the value Methodist sisters attached to it rather than the value attached to it by male Victorians or nonreligious women.[93] The evidence presented suggests that the sisters possessed awareness that piety and the "social concern" stemming from it could enable some middle-class Victorian women to negotiate a measure of power from men. This was the context for Ailie Gale's understanding of the role and obligations of God-centered women in the twentieth century.

2

Women Missionary Doctors
in Nineteenth-Century China

Empowerment-through-piety had prompted many nine-teenth century American churchwomen to organize auxiliaries, educate themselves and develop their leadership capabilities. It had induced the sisters to express their lives as a constant search to serve God and humanity to their optimal capacity. While the women did not express the explicit desire for career success, their ideals often rendered piety and professional accomplishment synonymous. Most, especially the wives of missionaries, had not been financially compensated for taking leadership positions; however, they too achieved a sense of self-respect and power normally attributed to paid professional American women.[1]

The cultivation-through-piety ideal's emphasis upon education led some Methodist women to pursue careers in medical work. In their capacity as doctors in the foreign field, the women could represent credibility, competence and power, while professing to serve God and humanity through their work as healers.[2] In this capacity, the women challenged middle-class Victorian notions of women's capabilities in the medical profession and in the professions as a whole.

Conversely, the women's self-representation reinforced American sup-porters' conceptions of Chinese inferiority, not only by the cultural su-periority reflected in their attempts at replacing Chinese medicine with their own, but by the very leadership skills that enabled them to challenge white patriarchal authority: despite their challenge to domestic notions of gender, the women still represented Western dominance over China. Thus, women who were successful at inspiring home field contributions for China encouraged the formation of complex bonds of challenge and constraint, among their supporters, the Chinese and themselves.

This chapter acknowledges the cultural imperialism inherent in the women's representations, and its role in creating perceptions of a special Sino-American friendship based upon Western dominance. While the issue of friendship based upon dominance is an oft-explored one, the chapter's central focus will be upon how single women medical missionaries found Chinese culture amenable to traditionally female concerns such as public health, and how their representations challenged middle-class Victorian, male-dictated notions of women in medicine.

The health of Chinese women and children was an issue of importance to American churchwomen, and they invested much energy and money into this interest. Part of this investment began through the work of Northern and Southern male-administered missionary boards, but with the first quarter-century of Methodist work in China, these boards had still not undertaken any formal or organized medical work, and the women desired very much to respond to the medical needs of Chinese women. As Methodist historian Walter Lacy has noted, it was the women's societies, rather than the male-administered Methodist Episcopal Board, that really began "medical work as a distinct and definite part of the development of the church."[3]

When married women missionaries in the field reported that social restrictions impeded Chinese, Hindu, and Muslim women from allowing male physicians to examine them, the response of women's boards was to build up the medical service as quickly as women doctors could be recruited.[4] The male boards gained momentum from the women's efforts and by 1910 there were 348 women physicians, 576 hospitals, and 1,077 dispensaries, gains reflected in the increased number of medical services for Chinese women and children.[5] A link between China, medical missionaries and women was established, and American female mission supporters would have a stake in it.

While it was the plight of Chinese women which concerned many American religious women, there was another element central to the appeal of support for women's medical work. The hospitals for women and children not only served Chinese women, but also offered professional opportunities to the American women doctors who administered them. Moreover, the work of medical missionaries was described to supporters just as women were taking their place in the medical field in America. Thus, the opportunities women physicians were provided in the foreign field are important in the context of American society's perception of women physicians amidst the evolution of medicine in America.

Post-1860s America was a trial period for women physicians, a time when women were "barred, for the most part, from men's schools," as historian Regina Markell Morantz-Sanchez notes.[6] While women made enormous strides during these decades, opening five major women's medical colleges in Philadelphia, New York, Baltimore, Chicago and Boston, they found themselves constantly forced to prove their superiority in the medical field.[7] Despite the excellent reputation of most of the women's colleges, prejudice against women in medicine persisted. For example, by 1893, only 37 of the 105 orthodox, male-established and administered medical institutions accepted women.[8] Much of this prejudice was owed to the middle-class Victorian emphasis upon the unique, innate traits of men and women.

During the 1850s, women were admitted into medical schools with the justification that medical science needed their feminine influence.[9] Indeed, the consensus among nineteenth and early-twentieth-century women doctors was that women had natural gifts as healers. These arguments led most advocates of women's fitness in the medical field, including women physicians, to argue that women were suited to practice by virtue of their innately feminine attributes, and that they would play a complementary, rather than equal role to their male counterparts.[10]

The belief in an innately feminine, "nurturing" contribution became an obstacle to women as the medical field evolved and "germ theory" narrowed the physician's perception of his patient's needs. With the increased focus upon patients' disease rather than their overall health and well being, the physician came to be increasingly defined in "scientific" rather than "social," or personal terms. Women would find themselves at a disadvantage within the medical profession precisely because they had been valued for their innate ability to nurture and treat the patient's "social context," rather than the disease.[11]

Methodist depictions of the work of female medical missionaries to China illustrate how the sisters' perception of traditionally female medical work contained emphases which countered certain important male-dictated, middle-class Victorian precepts. Portrayals of women physicians in missionary literature constitute an important, yet hitherto unrecognized example of female physicians' competence. The literature's importance is three-fold. Depictions of competent female missionary physicians helped in the overall struggle for women's legitimacy in the medical field. It provided women mission field supporters, including women doctors in America, with professional role models for identification, and it presented China, the host country, as a nurturing ground for female professionals.

One American medical doctor recalled that during her training at the Woman's Medical College of Pennsylvania from 1928–31, "one of the first things we were shown were the wonderful records of some of the medical mission women who had graduated."[12] That women doctors were inspired by the work of missionaries in the twentieth century is not surprising: missionary literature depicted women missionary physicians who left for China in the nineteenth century as early proponents of the concept that women could function competently in what was considered a male domain.

The deliberate goal of Sarah Hale, founder of the Ladies Medical Missionary Society, was not to encourage social recognition of a more public or professional sphere for women, or female physicians in general. Hale's editorship of the influential *Godey's Lady's book* allowed her to procure support from local Protestant churches for the founding of a society to finance the medical education of women desiring a missionary career. Concerned about the plight of "heathen women," Hale hoped that "medical women . . . might get access where Christians had never been allowed." Hale did not see medical work as a means to forge a more public existence for women because she saw no place for women in public. Yet, Hale, an advocate of education and property rights for married women in America, was a significant force for change.[13]

In 1851, when Hale first suggested the formation of a Ladies Medical Missionary Society, the notion had been too radical for acceptance and she was ridiculed mercilessly.[14] Helen Barrett Montgomery's 1910 account of the founding of Hale's Society, recalled the reason why: "There was that awful bogey of a woman going out of her sphere even for the saving of life."[15]

Mrs. Annie Gracey Ryder, a prolific chronicler of women Methodist achievements, was an educational missionary to India from 1861–67. Gracey returned home from India shortly before the WFMS became the first women's society to utilize Hale's society, sending out its first missionary, Dr. Clara Swain, to India in 1870. Gracey wrote many articles and tracts, and published four sketches between 1888 and 1891, while serving as General Executive Committee recording secretary of the WFMS Philadelphia Branch, which she had organized and founded in 1869.[16] Her earliest work, *The Medical Work of the Woman's Foreign Missionary Society* (1888), is a focus of this chapter because of Gracey's background as a member of the sisterhood which helped to build the missionary movement, a former missionary, and a proponent of the women's empowerment-through-piety ideal.[17]

Gracey's account of the work of female medical missionaries, beginning with the 1870 sailing of Methodist doctor Clara Swain to India, contributed favorably to arguments that women were not only adept at medicine by virtue of their intrinsic female morality—the "separate spheres argument," but also by their scientific know-how, competence and skill. In the introduction to her work, Gracey utilized a letter from a male doctor in China, Dr. Wiley, as a testimony to the high regard accorded women by their male coprofessionals. Wiley's letter first emphasized the conventional argument that women physicians were useful because of their unique ability to reach Chinese women and thereby achieve a "more powerful" moral result than that possible from "similar services rendered to the native men."[18]

Wiley continued with a statement which was later supported in Gracey's text with specific examples: female physicians in China had been able to establish hospitals of truly excellent quality. These hospitals had accomplished what Dr. Wiley himself would admit not having been able to realize:

> your lady physicians had commanded, by their skill and success, the recognition and respect of the male physicians of China, both of those who are acting as missionaries and of those who are having lucrative practice in the cities where many foreigners are found.[19]

Wiley's acknowledgement of the work of women by male doctors with "lucrative practices" is especially important: while Wiley does not give much detail regarding the identity of the male doctors, he suggests that they were enjoying the commercial rewards of their work, and from this secular (hence, presumably unbiased) perspective, could appreciate the competence of the women missionary doctors.

Gracey's text went on to describe the accomplishments of the women doctors, providing explicit evidence of how the women established successful hospitals in China. This was important because in nineteenth-century America, while women could work in women's dispensaries and women's hospitals in New York, Boston and Philadelphia, they were excluded from male-dominated hospitals by powerful professional medical associations and were often relegated to practicing from their homes.[20]

A powerful argument justifying this exclusion, and other forms of discrimination against professional women, was the Victorian ideal of female physical frailty and intellectual inferiority. According to historian Cynthia Epstein, this idea had a greater hold in America than elsewhere, and it was a strong factor preventing American women from entering professional life.[21] As discursive representation, rather than material reality, Gracey's narrative is an example of how missionary literature depicting women doctors in the field countered both the Victorian ideal of women's frailty and the rationale for female exclusion from practice in American hospitals.

Dr. Lucinda Combs, the first medical missionary sent by the WFMS to China in 1873, represented an exemplary female success story. While life had initially heaped some cruelty upon her, leaving her an orphan at an early age, Combs had managed to educate and support herself.

Her conversion experience had left her with the "constant thought" of "preparation for missionary work." Combs' first step toward fulfilling her goal of becoming a missionary was to enter a New York seminary. According to Methodist author Mary Sparkes Wheeler, at the seminary she was "unaided," relying completely upon herself. Despite her lack of assistance or support from outside sources, her "energy, tact and industry" kept her at the head of her classes. During vacations, others rested but Combs "toiled on unremittingly, as her motto was Excelsior," Wheeler noted, and "her perseverance and indomitable will easily overcame what to many would have seemed insurmountable obstacles."[22]

After graduating "with the highest honors" from a three-year course in the seminary, Combs became convinced of her calling as a physician, and set out for Philadelphia "without means to enter medical college." She had planned upon becoming an India missionary, having heard a lot "about the value of a medical education for lady missionaries." As Wheeler explained, Combs was "determined to secure such an education first . . . to leave nothing undone which would aid in qualifying her to the utmost for usefulness in her future work." She would support herself while attending college lectures, doing housework for a family, and with economic assistance from Hale's Ladies Medical Missionary Society. She graduated from the Woman's Medical College in Philadelphia and in 1873 was contracted by the ladies of the Philadelphia Branch for service as a China missionary.[23]

By the time of Combs's arrival, Peking, China's northern capital, was a prospering missionary field, with a hospital, under the control of the Parent Missionary Society. Medical work had begun there in 1861, and was continuing successfully, despite the fact that Chinese women were receiving little or no benefits from the efforts of the Methodist Episcopal Board.

Immediately upon arrival, Miss Combs insisted upon learning Chinese, despite the fact that medical missionaries were excused from waiting to become proficient in the language of the host country before beginning their practices, and instead allowed to work through interpreters. Combs worked hard at language study and, according to Gracey, made "such proficiency in the difficult language that at an early day she was able to do without an interpreter." While studying Chinese, Combs utilized her medical skills to make some home visits to Chinese women. Though her schedule was exhaustive, she was noted by another missionary observer as an "enthusiastic" worker who "enjoyed it heartily."

Combs's energetic work schedule was rendered even more impressive in the context of Gracey's depiction of the Chinese women Combs hoped to treat. Gracey described Chinese women in keeping with nineteenth-century missionaries' tendency to group together "third world women" as antithetical "other." Despite the reality of regional and national differences among the women, Gracey observed that middle and upper-class Chinese, like their Indian counterparts, were "secluded."[24]

It was precisely because these Chinese women confined to their homes, that Combs found her work difficult, noting that it was impossible for her to gain "access to the homes of the natives." Combs's problem prompted her to develop a plan which was exemplary for illustrating women missionaries' abilities to implement creative solutions to problems in the field: she asked for funds to construct a hospital building for Chinese women. Although she was in China for less than one year at the time, Combs took her plea for Chinese women to the Philadelphia Branch of the WFMS, requesting that they allow her "at an early date . . . to open a hospital."

At the meeting of the General Executive Committee in Philadelphia in May 1874, the appropriation was made for two thousand dollars toward the building of the Peking Woman's Hospital. The women mission field supporters responded quickly and affirmatively in support of the young woman doctor's efforts. By December of that year, Combs reported that the property was purchased. Within five years the woman's hospital was well on its way, complete with "spacious wards, the clinic rooms, dispensary rooms, waiting and bath, and all other necessary rooms," according to Gracey.[25]

As was typical of women missionary professionals, Combs's position as the sole woman doctor in Peking had allowed her the privilege of identifying the need for an institution, requesting and soon receiving the funds for its establishment, and overseeing the institution's development, in keeping with her specifications. In contrast to the limitations placed upon women physicians in America, this was quite a formidable accomplishment.

Combs's decision to construct dispensary rooms was reflective of women's social and nurturing role in the nineteenth-century American medical field, where dispensaries provided the needy with free medical care while affording supervised postgraduate training to young women doctors. In late nineteenth-century Baltimore, one such dispensary provided lectures on hygiene for women and girls, established the city's first distribution of clean milk to sick and needy babies and started the first public bath.[26] Combs had established an institution, which afforded American women doctors a decision-making role while simultaneously mirroring the efforts of American women doctors and representing the concerns of American women.

In her ability to raise money and have a hospital constructed, Combs's representation as a leader and achiever in medical work challenged white male doctor's patriarchal authority, and any middle-class Victorian claims that women were unfit for the professions; however, it simultaneously reinforced ideals of Western superiority over the Chinese. While Combs's hospital was under construction she came increasingly to be accepted into Chinese homes to heal "heathen" women and children. Gracey noted that Combs "prosecuted" her medical duties "in the midst of great difficulties, but with marked success in winning the hearts of Chinese women." Gracey described Combs's enemy as the dirt and lack of medical knowledge of her Chinese patients. In a language which typically categorized the Chinese as the antithetical "other," Gracey contrasted the cleanliness and beauty of the Methodist Board's and Women's Foreign Missionary Society buildings with the "tumble-down shanties" of the Chinese that were torn down to build them.[27]

While within five years Combs married a male missionary of the Parent Society, she continued to work as a missionary. According to Wheeler, in 1877, the couple moved to Kiukiang, where both continued in missionary work. Combs's replacement, Dr. Leonora Howard, took over the Peking Woman's Hospital in 1877.[28]

Gracey depicted Howard as similar to Combs in her ability to combat life's ordeals. The daughter of a Canadian physician, and a native of Syracuse New York, Howard was afflicted with many and "great" physical ailments. After graduating from the University of Michigan at Ann Arbor, her departure for the missionary field was almost impeded, "so frail was her health at times;" however, because "her heart had been given to the work," illness was overcome and she arrived in Peking on July of 1877.[29]

Despite her initial bad health, she was described by Gracey as a woman of "indomitable energy and perseverance." Howard's work in China never reflected the inability to combat physical weakness or fatigue. Rather, details regarding Howard's cases bear out her ability to maintain a grueling schedule as a physician by day and spiritual leader by night.

On a typical day she treated ward occupants, dispensary patients, and visited "downtrodden" outpatients living in destitute conditions, with no food, fire, or clothing. Howard's journals record that from July 1878 to March 1879, she treated 1,612 dispensary patients, 50 outpatients and 14 ward occupants. In the evenings Howard would hold religious services at the Peking Woman's Hospital.[30]

Howard's dispensary work paralleled women's early efforts in social medicine in America. She responded to patients' "most pressing needs," relating to all aspects of their existence: their physical and spiritual well being. Perhaps because Combs had earned the trust of Peking's poorest citizens, building a hospital and treating women and children in their homes, Howard reported that the Chinese were respectful of her treatment, expressing gratitude for even the smallest acts of kindness and care. Howard's perspective may have been an exaggeration, or wishful thinking, but its effect, the message that Peking's poor had proven a welcome ground for women's nurturing efforts in social medicine, bolstered American sisters' perception of women's capabilities as physicians. Moreover, according to Gracey, by 1879, Howard had established "a practice sufficient to occupy the time of two," and a reputation as a highly skilled physician. It was because of this reputation that Tientsin's Viceroy, the talented diplomat Li Hung-chang, formally requested that Howard visit his ill wife.[31] The turn of events which followed, intertwined with accounts of Li Hung-chang's willingness to enter into diplomatic relations with the United States, portrayed Dr. Howard, not only as a competent physicians, but as a vital player in Sino-American diplomatic relations.

Tientsin, a populous city, had been plagued by upheavals such as the Taiping and other rebellions since the 1850s. After the Tientsin Massacre of 1870, missionaries of other societies complained that even the appearance "of a foreigner on the street was the signal for the slamming of doors," according to Gracey. Many missionary societies reported that attempts to initiate missionary work in Tientsin between 1870 and 1879 had been a failure due to the pervasive antiforeignism among city residents. Methodists lamented that Tientsin's women, who numbered over two hundred thousand, were totally inaccessible.[32]

Due to the relationship between Dr. Howard and the man most responsible for putting down the Taiping Rebellion, Li Hung-chang, Gracey explained that the door to Tientsin would open. Li Hung-chang's Anhui Army had been the strongest anti-Taiping force during the 1850s. Born in Anhwei in 1823, Li was awarded the highest honors in the examination system by the age of twenty-four. Under the patronage of an eminent Chinese statesman, Li's career flourished, and he soon became an able military leader who would help stabilize the Ch'ing Dynasty despite massive internal rebellion.[33]

Li had benefited from the assistance of Western arms during the war, and together with other scholar-officials, had been involved in diplomatic negotiations with the United States since the 1860s. Li and others were part of the self-strengthening movement, whose tenets proclaimed that China could preserve Confucian values by learning from the West.[34]

By the 1870s, the encroachments of the imperialist powers became very threatening to China. Japan formally annexed the Liu-ch'iu Islands in April 1879 and Russia threatened the Ili region in Central Asia. In response to the reality that China was losing its tributary states to the imperialist powers, Li Hung-chang decided to take the advice of his

American friend, a family tutor, interpreter and private secretary named William Pethick, and seek the services of Ulysses S. Grant, who was scheduled to visit China during his world tour in 1879.[35]

When Grant and his wife visited Tientsin in 1878, they met with Viceroy Li Hung-chang and his wife, Lady Li. A Methodist missionary, Mrs. Davis, acted as interpreter for Mrs. Grant and Lady Li. Viceroy Li's meeting with the former president turned out favorably. Grant was perceived as a strong man of character, and Li, impressed that Grant had put down a major rebellion in his own country, asked Grant to appeal to Japan on behalf of China.[36]

Lady Li became seriously ill a short while after meeting with Mrs. Grant and Mrs. Davis, and according to Gracey, this deeply distressed her husband. Evincing the common female missionary allegation that most Chinese marital relations were shaped by the assumption that women existed only for the convenience of men,[37] Gracey commented that Viceroy Li possessed an unusual affection for his wife and he was "in great sorrow at the prospect of losing her." Initially, the Viceroy rejected the idea that his wife be seen by foreign doctors, as this was unheard of at the time, particularly among upper-class Chinese. He eventually consented, allowing a male physician from the London Missionary Society to provide Lady Li with medication to stabilize her condition. In order to effect a complete cure, however, the Viceroy's wife required closer contact with the physician and Chinese social ideas impeded this. In response to the suggestions of the United States Vice Consul and several male physicians, the Viceroy sent a special courier and later a steam launch to transport Dr. Howard to Tientsin.[38]

When Howard's remedies immediately cured Lady Li, the families of other high officials began requesting her medical services. Howard soon found herself torn between returning to Peking to serve the poor and staying in Tientsin to cure the well-to-do. She resolved this dilemma by looking toward "providence," which convinced her that another lady doctor could recommence her work with the poor, while in Tientsin there was a "wider field of usefulness which must be entered immediately, or the door might again be closed."[39]

The hospital for Peking's poor women would remain closed forever, unknowingly sacrificed by Howard for the opportunity she anticipated in Tientsin. Viceroy Li's gratitude to Dr. Howard was hearty, as interpreted not only by Methodist accounts but also by the secular press in America. According to Gracey, one Peking correspondent of the *New York Herald* described how Viceroy Li showed two noted American male doctors to the door, deciding instead to call in Dr. Howard, "whose skill he had heard as having effected some remarkable cures." *The Herald* described

Viceroy and Lady Li as generous in their expressions of gratitude toward Dr. Howard. They provided her with apartments for both a dispensary and surgery near the viceregal residence. There could be no doubt in the minds of readers that China was supporting American female forays into both the male domain of surgery and the female domain of social medicine, as the *Herald* explained:

> Here, with such an introduction as her connection with the family of the Viceroy gave her, opportunities for usefulness have rapidly multiplied, although overwhelming the devoted and skillful young doctor with arduous labor.[40]

Any reader of Gracey's work would have believed that it was due more to the efforts of Dr. Howard, than his faith in Grant, that Viceroy Li Hung-chang agreed to the Angell treaty of 1881. These accounts mention General Grant's attempt to resolve the dispute with the Japanese, but emphasize that Viceroy Li's decision hinged upon Dr. Howard's assurance to Lady Li that James G. Angell, President of the University of Michigan, Howard's alma mater, was a trustworthy man. The result of Howard's intervention was Li's agreement to limit Chinese right of free immigration to the United States as originally set in 1868 by the Seward-Burlingame Treaty.

In reality, Li Hung-chang's direct involvement with the treaty was limited. Li had indeed made some concessions to American exclusionists in 1879, when he accepted Grant's help in negotiations with Japan in exchange for agreeing to limit the emigration of Chinese laborers to the United States. But in 1880, the dispute over the islands continued and it was here that Li maintained his focus, leaving the foreign office and Li Hung-tsao to deal with the concessions delineated in what would become the Angell Treaty.[41]

As the decade passed, Viceroy Li grew angry at American mistreatment of Chinese immigrants in the United States, and the idea that China must protect foreigners on its soil. Subsequent acts restricting Chinese immigration infuriated him even more.[42] However, his hope for a special Sino-American friendship, and his attitude toward western women in medicine had provided a boon to the female Methodist missionary effort in Tientsin, and an inadvertent boost to women doctor's efforts to attain professional legitimacy in the American medical field.

Howard wrote to mission field supporters about the support provided by the Viceroy and his wife. Viceroy Li had donated a temple in the city for dispensary work, paying all the expenses himself, and contributing a sum of $2,700 to get the work going. Lady Li had provided Dr. Howard not only with apartments for work but monies to defray expenses. Gracey noted Lady Li's contribution of about $700 for medicine and her willingness to give more upon "presentation of the accounts." Appealing to churchwomen at home for more monies, Howard made sure to note the generosity of Lady Li:

> All this dispensary work, is done at a distance of two or three miles from our home. In time it will be necessary to erect a hospital for patients. Lady Li has contributed so liberally toward the dispensary work that it is hardly to be expected that she will be asked to give to a hospital. Others may contribute, but it may be necessary for the ladies at home to appropriate especially for this purpose.[43]

Gracey informed supporters at home that the "crowd of women always waiting to be attended to" at the dispensary rendered the opportunity for work by a woman doctor especially pleasing. The women in the home field doubtlessly found it appealing that the "leading statesman in China" was not only supporting a dispensary providing social medicine for women, but had donated one of the "finest heathen temples in Tientsin" to Howard for Christian work. As Gracey explained, the "Viceroy is an idolater for political reasons; but he is a man of great intelligence, and he appreciates Protestant Christianity."[44]

Women mission field supporters responded enthusiastically to the celebrity status of Howard, her triumphant efforts in Tientsin and her apparent help at securing such a favorable treaty for the United States. Their financial contributions immediately surpassed even those of Viceroy Li and his wife. According to Gracey, at the General Executive meeting of Columbus Ohio, one woman from Baltimore was "deeply interested in this great work," and made a donation of $5,000 dollars toward building what would become the Isabella Fisher Hospital in Tientsin. Dr. Howard would marry in 1884, but by as late as 1917, the ecumenical *Chinese Recorder and Missionary Journal*, reported that Howard's hospital, despite its limited amount of equipment, was uniquely modern, something that women could doubtlessly point to with pride.[45]

Howard had become a celebrity for both the "sympathetic" womanly skills and the "scientific" medical skills touted by other exponents of female professional competence. That these skills had been of what appeared to be extraordinary use in the highly public arena of United States diplomacy in the 1870s and 1880s doubtlessly enhanced the cause of women in the public sphere.

Importantly, Howard's success in establishing dispensaries and surgical facilities in Tientsin was purportedly owed to a distinguished Chinese statesman, a willing benefactor for women's medical needs and a supporter of Christianity. In summary, the story of the development of medical work in Tientsin reflects the inclination of women missionaries to portray China as a nation which welcomed, respected and supported professional Christian women. Historical accounts of the doctors at the woman's hospital at Foochow provide similar evidence in support of the advantageous opportunities for women in the China mission field. Gracey described Dr. Sigourney Trask as possessed of "quiet energy" and determination to succeed." These would serve her well in Foochow, where she would eventually earn a wide reputation for her "gentle, kind manner and unselfishness," typical of women's nurturing qualities, as well as for her skill as a physician.[46]

Trask was born in Pennsylvania in 1849. Like Luncinda Combs, she came upon hard times as a child. She lost her mother, but was raised by paternal grandparents who made sure that she attended the local Methodist church regularly. At the local church a pastor became impressed with Trask's potential, noting her "thirst for knowledge . . . superior mind," "studious habits," and "superior intellect." The pastor saw to it that she could attain an education appropriate for a woman whom "Providence . . . designed a more than ordinary sphere of usefulness" despite her limited financial means. He arranged the support of an anonymous donor, and Trask entered the Pittsburgh Female College, graduating with honors in 1870. Trask's decision to become a missionary and a doctor combined both elements of piety and self-actualization. She recalled "reading the Bible" in order to learn for what "purpose" God had sent her "into the world." Pondering each avocation in her mind, Trask noted:

> Nothing was satisfactory. All were exhausted. Teaching school, the last and more favorably considered, possessed an indefinable something which made even it not fully satisfactory.[47]

The decision to go to China as a missionary was a happy one because Trask realized that a definite direction lay ahead:

> it seemed as if I were in a new world. The new life had not come yet, but it was certainly a new phase in life to have something definite as an object.[48]

Trask decided simultaneously to become both a missionary and a doctor so that she might have a broader sphere of usefulness. Graduating in 1874 from Elizabeth Blackwell's Woman's Medical College of New York, she prepared to sail for China that year.[49] As a recent medical school graduate, Trask implied to friends that the decision to go to China as a medical missionary was an empowering one:

> The actual work of my life is to begin soon. I am so glad it is at hand! I do believe every feeling, faculty, and possibility of my nature is consecrated a living—I do not like to say sacrifice—a living energy to accomplish the mission God has given me among the Chinese . . . "Bound in spirit," Paul said: under bonds of the Spirit I go. This bondage is my liberty; the bonds are my joy and my strength.[50]

Dr. Trask was sent to Foochow by the New York branch of the WFMS in 1874. That city, with one of China's most important ports, contained a population of about one million. The Methodist church had begun its missionary work in Foochow in 1847. They provided Trask with a dispensary in a small building situated within the Methodist mission compound. Trask obtained some drugs from Hong Kong while awaiting shipments from America, and began attending to the women and children who came to her.

Unlike Doctors Combs and Howard, Trask was not immediately inclined to visit the Chinese in their homes, doing so "only in cases of necessity." She explained that when a foreigner would appear "at the average Chinese house . . . a multitude of men, women and children" would immediately take the house "by force." Like Combs, Trask appealed to the New York branch on behalf of the women and children, who came to her dispensary "with all manner of sicknesses," for a hospital for women.[51]

Within seven months from the date of her arrival, in May 1875, the General Executive Committee met and the Society responded to Trask's appeal by the appropriation of five thousand dollars, most of which was raised by the proceeds of a bazaar held by some of the New York and Brooklyn churches.[52]

While deciding upon a site and structure for the hospital, Trask attended to hospital matters, treating a total of 584 in-patients, performing thirty-eight surgical operations, and visiting patients in the city, nearby suburbs and surrounding country areas. Finally, by April 1877 the two-storied brick structure was completed, and a dedication ceremony was performed, with the United States Consul, several commissioners and all members of the foreign community present. In order to fulfill Trask's goal of serving all classes of Chinese, the Foochow Hospital for Women and Children was located on an island near the Min River, within a half-mile of seven native villages.[53]

Trask's accessibility and determination to serve all types of patients was emphasized by male Methodist doctors Baldwin and Beaumont of the

Parent Board at the hospital's inauguration in 1877, as each paid a tribute to Trask's past accomplishments and certain future successes. Baldwin noted Trask's impressive record for dispensary work and her treatment of "wives of mandarins and of wealthy persons in the city, as well as rich and poor in the country." With the new Hospital she would be able to continue this line of benevolent work. Beamont celebrated Trask's services to the poor and native women. At the close of ceremonies everyone cheered Trask on, applauding her success in carving "her enlarged sphere of action," according to Gracey.[54]

Trask's enlarged sphere of action included the medical domain commonly relegated to male doctors in the United States. During a Missionary Conference in Shanghai in 1877, Baldwin took the occasion to applaud, not only Trask's womanly proclivity for benevolent work, but also her technical skill. He made a commendatory speech recalling that Trask had been "asked to treat a case of dropsy that seemed so utterly hopeless" to him that he had gone "to the friends of the patient and told them that there was no hope." He was astounded when Trask was able to cure the patient. The story expressed a male doctor's view that Trask, a woman physician had been more competent at treating illness than he.[55]

At the same Shanghai Conference, Baldwin not only complimented Trask's medical skills but her administrative talents. He applauded her ability to establish a new hospital capable of receiving forty patients and treating them efficiently with all the necessary medicines and surgical appliances. Baldwin's approval of Trask's administrative skills and her superior capability at treating an illness were talents typically associated with male physicians. Gracey's reiteration of Baldwin's comments were a highly effective means of advertising Trask's successes, particularly given nineteenth-century American social conceptions of women's areas of competence in medicine.[56]

Trask's reports to missionary supporters in her society gave further evidence of her competence and skill. In her 1878 report, Trask noted that of the seventy-eight patients admitted into the wards within the past year, most had been surgical cases. Trask had performed amputations on arms and legs and removed tumors. No fatalities had resulted from the operations. Rather, Trask reported that confidence had grown: "there is now scarcely one who would not consent to an operation recommended, where formerly ten would refuse."[57]

Beginning in the nineteenth century and continuing into the twentieth, the supposition among the male-dominated American medical establishment was that women physicians were more inclined toward such traditionally female specializations as obstetrics, gynecology and pediatrics. By working with women and children, Trask was traditional, but her Trask's self-representation as a successful surgeon was an important validation of women missionary competence in a male-designated area of expertise.

Trask's competence in medicine was acknowledged, not only by patients but also by officials and the Methodist press in Foochow. She received both monetary support and praise from Chinese authorities. The smallest donations on the part of the Chinese were reported by Trask to the WFMS and mission supporters, and deemed reflections of Chinese confidence in Western women doctors. In 1878 Pao Heng, Acting Governor of Foochow and several other high officials of the province forwarded two hundred dollars to the United States Consul in support of Trask and her new hospital.[58] As further proof of Chinese recognition, Gracey shed light upon Chinese publications' admiration for Trask. Gracey cited the *Foochow Herald*, which described Trask as having "afforded invaluable medical and surgical relief to hundreds of Chinese women and children of all classes," who had benefited from her "professional skill."[59]

By 1878, Trask's success convinced the women's society that another woman doctor was needed to supplement the increasing work. Dr. Julia A. Sparr was born in Indiana in 1853. She had been converted at the age of ten during a revival. Thereafter she made her decision to devote herself to a missionary career as an adult. Her decision to study medicine stemmed from the wish to "enlarge the sphere of her usefulness." She graduated from the University of Michigan at Ann Arbor in 1877.[60]

Trask and Sparr divided their work between the hospital practice and the needs of the city and country residents. By 1879 the woman's society would raise the money for a new dispensary under the charge of Sparr. Located about three miles from the island Hospital, the Branch Dispensary quickly became popular. Within one year Sparr's new dispensary served 1,312 patients at the new location, over 100 patients more than the yearly average for Trask at the original dispensary on the Parent Board premises.[61] In 1884 Trask ended her ten years of service to marry and Sparr resigned the same year, soon after the arrival of Dr. Catherine Corey, the new physician appointed by the woman's society.[62]

Dr. Corey was a native of Indiana and a graduate the University of Michigan at Ann Arbor. Gracey's depiction of Corey best embodies the way in which a woman missionary doctor's pious motivations could subvert Victorian sphere demarcations. Corey was a skilled physician and her hospital reports were exemplary, providing detailed classification of the diseases treated and surgical operations performed since the incipiency of her work. The list of operations on her hospital reports included "cataract, amputation of the breast," corrections of corneal lacerations and cleft palate, according to Gracey.[63] When Corey's 1886 hospital report was submitted to, what Gracey referred to as "the high medical authority" in America, Corey received "unstinted praise." Revealing an essential motivation inspiring her chronicling of women doctors on the mission field, Gracey proudly argued that the highest medical authority's praise for Corey's report constituted proof of "women's fitness for the medical mission field."[64]

In addition, Gracey asserted that one leading American journal not only praised Corey's precision and surgical competence but her medical instruction at the hospital, which trained four Chinese female medical students. The journal identified the Foochow Hospital's course of study as "more advanced than that offered by many medical schools in our own country."[65] Most medical schools in America admitted only male students, therefore, Gracey's reiteration of the medical journal's opinion implied to readers that the female run Foochow Hospital was superior to many male-administered American medical schools.

Carrying forward the duties of the hospital and dispensary as well as the nursing duties formerly executed by both Trask and Sparr, Corey was a tireless worker. However, her performance was not without its personal disappointments. Despite the common nineteenth-century aversion to revealing one's feelings, Corey took the opportunity to express her frustrations. In so doing, she put her primary motivation into perspective, revealing the choices which had prompted her selection of a missionary career:

> My heart is sick and my ears sharpened instead of dulled by the pleading of the people. Had I simply wanted to practice medicine, because of the money in it, or the professional life, I would have stayed where both were offered me with more ease and larger emoluments. All the money in the missionary treasury could not keep me in China one year did not the love of Christ constrain me . . . this medical work is but a means to an end, and as such I must not let anything stand in the way of successful work.[66]

Motivated by piety, Dr. Corey had listed her alternatives in the United States, those of a medical career, money and professional life as secondary to religious service. Corey's recognition of the "emoluments" at home would have been understood by proponents of "Real Womanhood," who urged that women take up medical work rather than teaching or nursing because of the remunerations they could contribute to a family.[67] Supporters doubtlessly understood that Corey had been motivated by piety, rather than money, but Corey's statement was also an apparent rejection of the ideal of "True Womanhood" as well: she had not mentioned marriage as one of the forsaken "emoluments." In America, a woman doctor would not only have enjoyed money and a professional life but possibly marriage as well.[68] Thus, Corey's narrative was an expression of the empowerment-through-piety ideal in its suggestion that piety take priority over Victorian cultural presumption that all women marry and contribute either their household skills or their financial contributions to the home.

The professed goal of women missionary physicians in nineteenth-century China was to serve God and humanity. While their intention was not specifically to connect women with public life, the women's desire for optimal usefulness in their medical missionary work would prompt them to excel as professionals, take them out of their female sphere and suggest to nineteenth-century Americans that women physicians could function as competently as men.

Women missionary doctors in China represented images of privileged female empowerment in four ways: firstly, they found avenues of fulfillment by expanding upon the legacy of female interest in social medicine, enabling women in the home field to contribute monies toward programs that reflected a typically female approach. Secondly, while women missionary doctors worked with women and children, they also challenged the idea that women should be restricted to typically female subspecializations, such as pediatrics, obstetrics and gynecology, and subservient roles within the profession. The women's correspondence to the home field, as reflected in Gracey's narrative, enhanced their credibility in the scientific realm of surgery and in their ability to raise money for the construction and administration of hospitals.

Thirdly, while Gracey sometimes described the women doctors as physically weak, their representation as competent, hard working physicians challenged the Victorian assumption of women's inability to conquer physical and emotional obstacles. Finally, the women inspired readers to take an interest in international issues, by linking Chinese officials' support and political developments, to the problems missionaries attributed to Chinese women.

Women missionary representations were not only complex because they combined conventional garb with unconventional messages, but because they challenged conceptions of the subservient "place" of white women while reinforcing conceptions of the inferiority of "third world women." Consequently, while the women subverted their American sisters' conceptions of domestic order, theirs was not a wholesale attempt to change a hierarchical order based upon Western perceptions of dominance over China. Moreover, nineteenth-century women missionary doctors' representations as competent physicians and leaders in the China field were enhanced by their positing of Chinese culture, homes, women and children as the uncivilized "other" to be liberated by Western women.

In conclusion, when we view nineteenth-century medical missionaries through their representations within the American social and cultural context, it is apparent that their conservative garb belied unconventional messages, and that many of their images challenged as well as reinforced Victorian ideals. It is impossible to determine whether American supporters in the home field were drawn more to the representations of the women's challenge to patriarchal authority, or to their conservative garb and status as privileged white women; however, when assessing the roots of the "Special Sino-American" friendship, it is important to consider the aspects of both challenge and constraint characterizing Methodist women's discursive self-representation and images of China.

Part II

3

Dr. Ailie Gale: The American Setting

Dᴜʀɪɴɢ ᴛʜᴇ ᴄᴏᴜʀsᴇ ᴏғ ʜᴇʀ ғᴏʀᴛʏ-ᴛᴡᴏ ʏᴇᴀʀs ᴀs ᴀ Cʜɪɴᴀ ᴍɪs-
sionary, Dr. Ailie May Spencer Gale's correspondence to supporters
painted a self-portrait of both tradition and modernity. Americans de-
sirous of a larger public role for women could find Gale's representation
as a successful, independent woman physician appealing. This was so
because while twentieth century women doctors in America attempted to
gain recognition in a male-dominated medical field, Gale self-confidently
reported successes treating Chinese patients, appreciation for her work,
and vast administrative and surgical accomplishments.

Conversely, Gale appealed to supporters who championed a more
traditional woman's role. Gale's letters reflected her life as a wife, mother,
homemaker and hostess: Ailie and Francis Gale raised four children, and
Gale depicted her marriage as the companionate ideal admired by many
in post-Victorian America.[1] This dual representation helps explain an
aspect of Gale's connection to home field supporters.

Through her image as both modern and traditional, Gale forged a
bond with supporters that enabled her to explain events in China and
raise money for her host country. Gale's work in China coincided with
important developments there.[2] Years of fast-paced turbulence were intertwined with vital issues pertaining to the organization and international
status of the Chinese nation: civil war, Sino-Japanese War, Sino-American
alliance, and Communist victory.

During these important years, Gale was, like many women missionaries, at the crux of a complex relationship binding mission field supporters
to the Chinese in her daily life.[3]

This relationship was partly based on the discursive framework of
Western dominance, but also upon ideas of intercultural friendship and
cooperation. As a white woman and representative of an imperialist
power, Gale was complicit in the structure of Western domination.
More directly, her attempt to impose Western ways on a China struggling for self-determination against Western and Japanese dominance,

supported the notion of Western and white supremacy. In addition, her self-representation as a successful physician, hospital administrator and surgeon, offered supporters and the Chinese a model of white, rather than Chinese female success in the medical field. Consequently, one can argue that Gale challenged American notions of the legitimacy of white male superiority in the American medical field while undermining the power of the Chinese. By contemporary feminist standards, which rightly assert the notion that "feminism is about the empowerment of all women and change in the conditions of all women's lives," then Gale is not a feminist and does not attempt to challenge or transform existing social structures.[4]

On the other hand, Gale's writings sheds light upon how a Western woman's struggles against patriarchal order were entwined, not only to the conditions of other oppressed groups but to a woman's own self-understanding. Gale's predilection for traditional ideas such as "humaneness" in medicine, concern for the whole patient, (as opposed to the study of disease alone) and conceptions of "social concern" stemmed from nineteenth-century female Protestant social values that had been associated with, not only traditional, but sphere-enlarging impulses.[5] These complex understandings are what linked Gale and many other women missionaries to the Chinese, as well as to their American sisters in the home field.

Gale handled nearly all of the family correspondence to the home field from 1909–50, thus helping to shape supporters' views regarding events in China.[6] Moreover, like many women Methodist missionaries, Gale maintained an active schedule of speaking engagements while on furlough in America from 1913–15, 1922–23, 1930–32, and 1938–41, thus solidifying bonds established through correspondence.

An important aspect of Gale's relationship with supporters hinged upon the financial resources necessary to keep missionaries in the foreign field and the dissemination of information resulting from this need. Methodist churches in the United States were given the option of supporting either foreign districts, conferences, institutions or families in the field in accordance to what was known as the Parish Abroad Plan. In exchange for what was monetarily entitled, the special Parish Abroad Assignment, the Board would provide the church with a close association with the missionaries, promising them regular correspondence with an educational value, an "opportunity to establish a direct and very real connection between" the church and the work "on the foreign field." As the Methodist Board explained to one California church supporting the Gales in the 1930s:

> Missionaries are asked to write quarterly letters to their supporting constituency. When a church assumes the support of a missionary it is hoped that

a close and personal relationship will be established between the church and its missionary which will be mutually helpful. Letters from the home church to the missionary, expressing sympathetic interest in the work, bring to him courage and cheer, while his letters will keep the home church informed regarding the progress of the work, its problems and opportunities.[7]

General letters reporting the overall progress of mission work would not merely be confined to the church or churches participating in the Parish Abroad Plan. It was common for churches to use segments from missionary letters for publication in their weekly or monthly bulletins.[8] In addition, the missionary in the field would make copies for the various organizations affiliated with the church and contributing to the missionary's work. For example, in 1923, the Gale family was supported by only one church, yet Ailie Gale calculated that the twelve copies she had made of her first impressions of the Tunki mission field would reach a total of sixty-three different groups of people.[9]

Gale employed several means for circulating her letters among supporters. Many of Gale's "Dear Friend" letters were circulated through Priscilla Burtis, an active home field missionary worker and parishioner at the Simpson Church, in Brooklyn, New York, with whom she maintained a lifelong friendship.[10] Often recipients of Gale's quarterly letters were given a list of names so that they might make facsimiles and forward copies to the next name on the list. By 1924 Gale had 60 addresses on her mailing list, and in 1935, 125.[11] In addition, due either to the efforts of Gale or her supporters, quarterly letters occasionally reached local newspapers like the *San Francisco Examiner*, the *New York Advocate*, the *World Outlook* and other Methodist publications scattered throughout the United States.[12]

Gale's audience was made broader by the efforts of the Methodist Episcopal Board. Like all existing Protestant Boards, the Methodist Episcopal Board of Missions circulated the letters of many of their missionaries.[13] During the 1920s, the Board would extract information from missionary correspondence and send publicity newsletters to the larger group of contributors to the Methodist Episcopal Board of Foreign Missions. Women missionaries such as Gale penned an important segment of these extracts.[14]

As a member of her household, Gale was a beneficiary of the Parish Abroad Plan. From 30 December 1910 until 1925, the Simpson Church, in Brooklyn, New York, had raised the total $2,100 necessary for the annual support of the Gale family in the mission field.[15] In 1925 the Methodist Board conducted a study to determine the average amount necessary to support a family in China. On the basis of its conclusion, the Board upgraded the Gale's family allotment by $900, assigning the remainder of the support to a church in Twin Falls, Idaho.[16]

Gale was considered an inspirational magnet for drawing this additional support from the Twin Falls Church. The Board believed that details of her medical accomplishments, rather than Reverend Francis Gale's evangelical work, would draw the monies. Indeed, when the Methodist Episcopal Board initially informed the Gales of the Twin Falls Church's support, they also provided her husband, Reverend Francis Gale with a clear directive: That his correspondence make reference to his wife's medical work. According to the Twin Fall church's World Service treasurer, Mrs. Rounds, the yearly contribution of parishioners had previously been less than $600. It was expected that "the privilege of designating" the church's money toward Dr. Gale, "a missionary physician" would "result in an increase of interest," and consequently of money.[17]

In 1929, events further testified to Gale's effectiveness in communicating details of China medical work to supporters. When Mrs. Rounds moved to California, she established a connection to the Mission Hills Church, in San Diego, and saw to it that the Gales were given an additional support of $200 by her new church. This support, too, was contingent upon the assurance that the church might receive quarterly letters regarding Gale's medical work in China.[18]

As Americans experienced the hardships of the worldwide depression, churches continued to raise monies, but the sums grew smaller. In response to reductions in the total sum raised annually by the Simpson Church, smaller shares of support were taken up by a variety of other churches, including, by 1934, the Nevada City and Sierra County Parish, in Sacramento District of California.[19] The spreading out of smaller sums of support among more numerous churches meant that Gale's letters would reach more destinations and that news of her medical work would reach a broader and larger audience.

In 1934 the Methodist Episcopal Board of Missions informed the Gales that their ties to the Simpson Church would be subjected to the change in policy in effect for the entire Central China Mission. The Gales' support would be given to the Illinois Conference, a group of churches. Upon hearing of news of this change in 1934, Gale protested the Board's decision to assign them to "some church" with no prior knowledge of the family's history.[20] By 1935 when the decision was finalized, Gale noted that a "tie that had been so precious" had been severed. She wondered how she could "pray for something so indefinite" as the "Illinois Conference" of which "we know nothing."[21] Gale was doubtlessly aware that the same held true for Simpson parishioners, who would no longer have a long history of association with the new missionary family they were supporting.

Despite this emotional setback, Gale's ties to supporters became more extensive, as she would not only correspond with the Illinois Conference, but continue to write to the Simpson Church and the growing numbers of supporters on her address list.[22] In late 1948, two years before the Gales' departure from Communist China, the Methodist Board would return to the system of assigning one church to each missionary family and assign the Gales to a North Carolina church with 1,350 parishioners. This meant that Gale would share her impressions of the Chinese Communists with the new church, as well as the supporters she had corresponded with in the past.[23]

The Methodist Board directed Gale's far-reaching correspondence network; however, her correspondence went beyond Parish Abroad Assignments. There were individuals and organizations in the United States who independently provided Gale with regular contributions of money, children's clothing, Christmas gifts and medical supplies. Gale maintained correspondence with Methodist and other Protestant Churches, Sunday Schools, Junior Leagues, Ladies Aid Societies and women's groups. The supporters were spread across the United States: Oak Park and Evanston, Illinois; Oakland, Santa Fe, Watsonville, Long Beach, Los Angeles and Pasadena, California; Long Branch, New Jersey; Portland, Oregon, and Dennison, Michigan. From these diverse locations, individuals that she regularly corresponded with, and those to whom she had never written, sent gifts and monies to the Board for Gale, or directly to her address in China.[24]

Gale's correspondence influenced an immeasurable audience during the critical years of Sino-American alliance during World War II. From the late 1930s to the mid-1940s, Gale inspired supporters to give to a variety of Methodist Episcopal Board related relief organizations.[25] Moreover, Gale was one of many missionaries who indirectly assisted President Franklin D. Roosevelt's efforts to encourage Americans to contribute monies for China through the American Red Cross.[26]

While it is impossible to ascertain the exact amount contributed by Americans to these organizations, one thing is clear: Gale repeatedly encouraged and thanked her readers for contributing to the International Relief Committee, the American Red Cross, and the Methodist Committee for Overseas Relief.[27]

Despite Gale's status with supporters, and her presentation as a diligent professional, she represented a paradox common to most female spouses: she was never a formally appointed, salaried missionary. Apart from Reverend Francis Gale's salary and family allotment, she would never receive a stipend and the Board had never formally required her to engage in any work whatsoever. The arrivals and departures of the Gale family were noted in missionary periodicals, but the wife of Rev. Francis Gale was simply referred to as Mrs. F. C. Gale, rather than doctor, and because she was not legally an appointed missionary, she is conspicuously absent from the influential, ecumenical periodical, *The Chinese Recorder*. Moreover, for the five years that Gale worked for the Shanghai American School (1927–32), her $800 per year annual salary was deducted from the Gale family's $3,000 household salary.[28]

It was not surprising that Gale had committed herself to a lifetime of unpaid social activism. It was common knowledge among missionaries that most wives nearly always chose to undertake duties in the field despite the lack of pay. In part, this had to do with the strength of the empowerment-through-piety ideal, or the women's belief in the need to serve the Lord through social activism. As one male missionary put it: "no woman with consecration enough to come to the field will be content to be wholly idle after reaching it."[29] One female West China missionary, Florence Manly, noted that if a missionary wife was the type who wanted a strictly home-based existence, she would be most unhappy in China. As Manly observed, most wives were educated women who did not find that it took "all their time and energy to look after their husbands."[30]

While the family salary represented the male missionary's compensation for work, wives benefited from the lower cost of living in China. A salary from America went far, freeing the married woman from the domestic work that would have been her fate in her home country, and affording her an entire staff of Chinese servants. Women missionaries' reliance upon the Chinese for the mundane tasks associated with traditional Victorian domesticity enforced notions of female Western superiority while subverting patriarchal authority. Women rationalized this contradiction by expressing happiness at the opportunity to utilize their talents while providing a livelihood for the Chinese staff in their employ.

Ultimately, the absence of a formal salary did not mean that a missionary wife was any less active a worker than her formally appointed husband. On the contrary, monetary adjustments in China meant that she had more opportunity for creative, social activist tasks outside the home than she would have had in America.

The absence of a salary for married women may appall contemporary readers; however, it would not have precluded early twentieth-century American women readers' identification with female missionaries as role models of empowerment. Professional women in America were paid less than men in nearly all fields. Moreover, the level of pay was not as important an issue as it is now in a full-blown market economy. Most women sought challenge, independence, autonomy and accomplishment, all attainable in the mission field.[31]

Historian Peter Filene has argued that it was the mostly upper-middle-class woman who identified with these nonmonetary rewards. However, what Filene terms "salvation by work," was a secular counterpart for empowerment-through-piety, and was characteristic of many women missionaries, most of whom were of not of upper-middle-class origins.[32] Gale believed that "money is only a small part of life" and that "there are so many fine things left." Further, she had not applied this belief solely to women. When her three male children reached adulthood, Gale suggested that each pursue a career that they believed they were well suited for, as opposed to one with lucrative financial rewards.[33]

Gale's upbringing was typical for fostering the assumptions that would underlie a career based upon nonmonetary measures of success. American mission supporters could relate to Gale's professional achievements because they represented the realization of a desire for social activism initially inspired within nineteenth-century American Protestant female culture. Gale's early childhood and young adulthood provides a microcosmic view of the empowerment-through-piety ideal in the late nineteenth century, thus illustrating the basis for one missionary's ability to create relationships with her twentieth-century home field supporters.

Ailie May Spencer's childhood and the fundamentalist brand of Methodism of her circuit rider, preacher/dentist father, laid the foundation for her eventual espousal of the empowerment-through-piety ideal. Ailie Spencer's father, Moses Harrison Spencer, and his Scotch-Irish wife, Elizabeth, had traveled to Montana by stagecoach from the east coast during the mid-1800s. Born in North Carolina, Moses Spencer was both a healer and a religious man, a product of both Northern and Southern Methodist culture. He had studied dentistry and been a chaplain during the Civil War. Most of Moses Spencer's days were spent on horseback, riding circuit with dental instruments on one side of his saddle and his bible on the other.[34]

In Bozeman, Montana, in 1878, Ailie May Spencer was born into a spartan regime ruled by a father intolerant of any form of dissent. Both parents insisted that Ailie Spencer and her brother John pray daily and attend church regularly. Household edicts forbade any form of fun or game-playing, emphasizing the importance of education with equal vigor. Hence, Ailie Spencer's dominoes could only be utilized for the mind-enriching task of simulating the track of a locomotive, Bible and schoolbooks were mandatory, and fiction books were prohibited.[35]

Parental emphasis upon learning dictated that Ailie Spencer take the option of higher education when she came of age in 1898. By the time she was five, the family had relocated to Pueblo, Colorado and at the age of twenty, Spencer attended nearby Colorado College, in Colorado Springs.[36] The family's support was limited: while providing encouragement, they could not contribute financially, and this forced her to work as housekeeper and cook to continue her schooling. Despite financial hardship, while at Colorado College she decided to prolong her education and aim to be both a physician and a missionary. By 1901, critical events in her life would facilitate this transition: Spencer graduated from college and both her parents passed away.[37]

The death of her parents led to increasing financial strains, but Spencer managed to continue her education and in 1901 she was admitted to San Francisco's Cooper Medical College.[38] Spencer was nearly penniless during her three years at Cooper, surviving on raisins, fruits and vegetables donated by friends, and twenty dollars per month from her share of the rental of the family home in Pueblo, Colorado. While at Cooper, she joined the Student Volunteer Movement, pledging herself to the evangelization of the world in one generation.[39]

Spencer earned extra money by speaking in various churches on behalf of the Student Volunteers; however, most of her spiritual work was done without monetary compensation. In 1902, prior to the start of her term at Cooper, she had served as a missionary to New Mexico Indians. In 1903 she worked for the Epworth League and was secretary of a chapter of the Student Volunteers at the nearby University of California at Berkeley. During her remaining two years, she presided as vice-president, and later president of the Student Volunteers.[40]

Like the many women who worked to build women's missionary societies, Spencer was unrestrained by Victorian mores against public speaking. She spoke confidently because she believed that prayer would bring guidance from the Holy Spirit, who would make sure that her "words will be the right words."[41]

Among the circle of female Student Volunteers, there was a consensus that Spencer was "talented" and "accomplished," and that she was destined for more than marriage. In 1903, the Epworth League Department of Spiritual work described Spencer's as "the most admirable piece of work of any campaigner." She was deemed a vital force for "interesting the people of the Pacific Coast in missions." While presiding over one student volunteer meeting, Spencer met Francis Gale, then a young theology student at Berkeley, and by 1905, they would become engaged.[42]

Some women in her Student Volunteer group feared that Spencer's great future might be stifled by the "encumbrance" of her 1905 engagement, and prospective marriage to Francis Gale.[43] However, Spencer and her future spouse both believed in what I have termed: women's empowerment-through-piety. "Womanhood" was often a topic of Francis Gale's Sunday sermons, and Spencer described herself as happy with the "vital truths" he held on the topic.[44] Given what she believed was their shared conception of a woman's role, Spencer and Francis Gale married in 1905.

Although Francis Gale had applied to the Board of Foreign Missions while still a student at Berkeley, the board secretary suggested that he wait until after graduation. After the Gales married in 1905, the couple held a pastorate in California for three years. It was Ailie Gale who reminded her husband that they should be on their "way to China."[45] They would have two sons by the time of their commission to the China field by the Methodist Episcopal Board of Missions in 1908.[46]

Dr. Gale sought a career as a medical missionary for the purpose of winning souls for Christ, rather than for professional gain. In 1905, after receiving her medical degree, she did not take her state board examinations.[47] She had been convinced that she would use her medical skills on the mission field, rather than in America. Her actions proved prophetic, as she would be leaving behind a medical field which offered an inauspicious future for women physicians.

Gale's 1905 graduation from medical school in America had coincided with the onset of what many historians depict as bleak years for the progress of women in medicine. These were years in which, as historian Regina Markell Morantz-Sanchez observes, "nineteenth-century beach-heads were surrendered and lost to the champions of male backlash and institutional discrimination."[48] In 1902, three years before Gale's graduation, there were 1,200 women medical students in the United States, while in 1926, there were only 992 out of a total of 18,840. Gale was one of Cooper Medical College's 4 women graduates in 1905. By 1908, the number of female graduates at Cooper had gone down to 2.[49] As the decades progressed, women physicians became even scarcer. The numbers of women doctors did not reach 1910 levels until 1950, and there would be no dramatic increase until 1970.[50] Thus, as bastions of a slowly shrinking group of women medical professionals, Gale and other women missionary doctors can be viewed as role models for American women for more than the first half of the twentieth century.

When women missionaries wrote of the increasing opportunities for women physicians in China, and presented evidence of optimism concerning women in the China medical field, this information starkly contrasted with the American scene. The decrease in the numbers of women in medicine reflected a narrowing of opportunity for women physicians practicing in the United States. Inextricably tied to this was a discrimination against women medical students and physicians. In the twentieth century, the American Medical Association (AMA) would establish exclusive and demanding standards in order to hold the medical profession to a higher degree of competence, while simultaneously weakening the position of women in medicine. Women's schools were unable to obtain the financial backing necessary to purchase the expensive forms of technology which would meet the higher standards required by the AMA. Consequently, most closed their doors by the turn-of-the-century. The existence of coeducational schools such as Cooper Medical College, did not ameliorate these difficulties, as quotas limited the numbers of women accepted into their institutions.[51]

The quest for higher standards would lead to the increasing necessity for hospital training among medical school graduates and to another obstacle for women. Internships had not been an important aspect of medical training in the nineteenth century: Consequently, they had not been a concern for women. As each decade of the twentieth century progressed, however, state medical boards came increasingly to require internships, and hospitals would make it more and more difficult for women to obtain them.

Thus, Gale's conviction that she would not practice medicine in the United States was likely owed to her awareness of the difficulties for women in obtaining hospital internships. Gale had been one of only eight out of a total of seventy-five male and female students that had entered Cooper with a four year-degree, and she had specialized in surgery while there. However, the extent of her postgraduate practical experience had consisted of accompanying a male doctor on rounds.[52]

With each passing decade, the American public became increasingly aware of the existing difficulties for women physicians. For example, one 1923 New York Times article reported the protests of 35 female medical students representing the College of Physicians and Surgeons at Bellevue Medical College, Long Island College Hospital and Flower Hospital Medical College. They "launched a movement by which they hope to open the doors of the hospitals" of that city wide enough for women to become interns.[53] By the 1930s, 5,000 male graduates would find 6,000 internships available, but 250 women medical school graduates were forced to compete for 185 internships. Ironically, medical schools justified their quotas limiting women students by citing female graduates' inability to obtain an internship. On the other hand, hospitals justified their unwillingness to give women internships by pointing out that there were not enough female medical school graduates to warrant the construction of women's living quarters in hospitals.[54]

In light of supporters' knowledge of the difficulties experienced by women physicians in America, depictions of the medical feats of women like Gale offered the opportunity for an appealing corrective. Gale's representation of her professional successes would be inversely proportional to the increasing difficulties for women doctors in the United States. Clearly, this was a reciprocal relationship: Gale benefited from contributions, and supporters benefited from their perception that they were responsible for the accomplishments of a woman physician. As such, Gale's success depended upon her ability to maintain her positive self-representation and enhance her credibility among supporters.

The following chapters detail Gale's work in Nanchang, Tunki, Shanghai, Nanking and West China on the basis of these queries: How was Gale's medical work tied to the empathetic bond she cultivated with supporters? How was the relationship between Gale and supporters reciprocal, and what did Gale give supporters in exchange for their monies? How did Chinese recognition of Gale's professional status enhance her credibility? How was Gale's credibility linked to those individuals who validated her medical work; and how did this lead her to interpret events in China?

4

The Notable Nanchang Woman Physician

GALE, HER HUSBAND, TWO-YEAR-OLD SON OTIS SPENCER, AND SIX-month-old son Lester Sinclair, arrived in China in 1908, an auspicious time. With the death of the Empress Dowager, China was on the threshold of a revolution that would usher in many new beginnings, most of which promised the espousal of Western ways. The Ching Dynasty's Manchu rulers had governed China since 1644, but now were discredited by their inability to implement the reforms demanded by increasing numbers of educated, nationalistic Chinese. The questioning of the "mandate of heaven," or the Manchu emperor's right to rule, the abolition of the ancient examination system in 1905 and the weakening of Confucianism (with its insistence upon "the three bonds"), all dealt a blow to traditional ideas based upon hierarchical order.[1]

Missionaries perceived these changes as suggestive that the Chinese were inclined to accept democracy and Christianity as legitimate alternatives to the discarded ways. Female Nanchang missionary Welthy Honsinger noted that "all . . . insignia of rank . . . are filling curio shops. The Governor will never ride forth in state to my lodge house preceded by his red umbrella." In Nanchang, a Chinese pastor who had previously not been allowed into the homes of officials, found that after the 1911 revolution he had the respect of the entire community.[2] Medical missionaries were especially optimistic.[3]

In response to the North Manchurian Plague of 1910 and 1911, the new Republican government granted its official recognition of Western medicine. By 1913, official authorization was also given to anatomical dissection.[4] These milestones would have an impact upon female physicians.

With the Manchu abdication of 1911, two factors made the China medical field a particularly promising one for women doctors like Gale: missionary optimism about Chinese acceptance of Western medicine, and awareness that the China medical field was severely understaffed.[5] As one of about 450 medical missionaries in China during the 1910s, Gale had the good fortune of arriving in Nanchang in time to experience the confluence of these forces.[6]

In 1909, when the Gales arrived in Nanchang, the capital of Kiangsi, they found three Methodist institutions that would soon offer Dr. Gale professional opportunities: the Stephen L. Baldwin Memorial Girls' School, with a home and teachers' buildings and two hospitals, the Board's Nanchang General Hospital and the Women's Foreign Missionary Society's Women and Children's Hospital.

The Methodist Episcopal Board's medical work in Nanchang began in 1902 with a small building for ten inpatients and an outpatient clinic. By 1909 the Board appointed Dr. J. G. Vaughan Superintendent of medical work. Soon Vaughan was commissioned to purchase land for buildings for the envisioned Nanchang General hospital and, with no other Western physician available, the Methodist Board's hospital came under Gale's direction.

While the Methodist Board did not officially acknowledge Gale's position in any of its publications or annual reports, Gale's correspondence indicates that she served as chief administer at the Nanchang Hospital until 1922. Until 1920, she was the only physician for the hospital of thirty beds and two outside dispensaries.[7] That year, after many persistent requests, she finally found an associate Chinese physician to work alongside her.[8]

Nanchang's first girls' school, then known as "Protecting Spirit," had been built by a WFMS missionary in 1902. By 1908 there were 54 girls enrolled in the school, and by 1913, the year that it was turned over by the WFMS to the Methodist Episcopal Board, it was known as the Baldwin School, and it enrolled 120 pupils from the kindergarten to middle school levels. Gale was the school's physician beginning in 1910. Consequently, after two years in China, Gale provided medical services for both the WFMS and the MECB.[9]

Dr. Ida Kahn, a missionary and United States–educated Chinese doctor who developed an excellent reputation among the Chinese in Kiangsi Province, began medical work for Nanchang women. Kahn and her colleague, Dr. Mary Stone had been legendary as the first Chinese women to open a hospital in China. Both had been students at the WFMS educational missionary Gertrude Howe's boarding school (est. 1872), the first for girls in the Yantze Valley. Gertrude Howe had arranged for both Kahn and Stone to enter the medical school at Ann Arbor, Michigan in 1892.[10] In 1896, the two women graduated and returned to their native Kiukiang. A few years later, Kahn and Stone established the Elizabeth S. Danforth Memorial Hospital in their home city.[11]

Dr. Kahn left Kiukiang in 1903, when the Nanchang gentry requested her medical services in their city after learning of her successful treatment of the wife of a Kiukiang high official. That year the Nanchang gentry provided Kahn with land and the funds to open a dispensary. In 1906, Kahn transferred the deeds to the dispensary building, and the land it was situated on, to the WFMS, who put her on their payroll. However, Kahn required more than the WFMS stipend to fulfill her dream of building a hospital for women. In 1908, the year that Gale arrived in China, Kahn and Howe left for the United States to raise money for a hospital building on the site donated by Nanchang gentry.[12] Kahn raised some money, then remained in the United States to complete an A.B. degree at Northwestern University. Kahn's departure had left an opening for women's medical work in Nanchang and Gale filled that opening until Kahn's return.

Gale took charge of the medical work for both men and women of Nanchang in 1909. Beginning in 1910, Gale's days were spent shuttling between the Baldwin School, the Methodist Episcopal Board's Hospital (adjacent to the oval mission compound and the three story building in which she and her family lived) and the Woman's Dispensary, located thirty minutes walking distance from the Board's hospital. Gale handled most phases of medical work at the three locations, performed surgical operations and made housecalls to patients of all classes, financing treatments for the poor with fees to upper-class patients.[13]

Like most Western doctors, Gale encountered some opposition from the Chinese and her medical efforts in Nanchang were not uniformly successful. Chinese patients often were brought to foreign doctors only after their condition had caused extreme deterioration. In both her correspondences to family and supporters, however, Gale chose to ignore the disappointing medical cases and the resistance of the Chinese and instead focus on her successes.

Supporters were told that Nanchang offered Gale the opportunity of performing complex and unusual surgical procedures that would have tested the abilities of the most competent of surgeons. For example, Gale performed an intricate surgical procedure on one twenty-eight-year-old man who had had necrosis of the jaw. She removed a malignant growth from a woman with breast cancer, then used the skin of the woman's son to graft the affected area. Gale described each patient as grateful enough to bring ill friends back to the Nanchang General Hospital for treatment by Gale. By 1919, Gale reported that the hospital was so full she was forced to turn patients away.[14]

Gale informed the home field of Chinese officials' appreciation for her surgical skills. A copy of a 1918 proclamation, forwarded to supporters in the United States, described Nanchang's Chief of Police, Yien Ngen-yung's praise for Gale: she was "an American emminent doctor of medicine. Since she has taken charge of Nanchang Hospital all her surgical operations have been very successful."[15]

Yien's apparent admiration for Gale's surgical skills contrasted with most American women physicians' relegation to the traditionally female fields of pediatrics, public health, teaching and counseling. Historians have argued that many women doctors in America confined themselves strictly "to the health problems of women and children because they hoped to raise the moral tone of society through the improvement of family life" and because they did not wish to antagonize their male counterparts.[16] Gale's correspondence to supporters depicted a successful foray into the scientific, male-dominated realm of surgery. In this realm, Gale had not only reported attaining success but also gaining the recognition of Chinese authorities, thus strengthening her credibility with American supporters. Gale also addressed those readers who were comfortable with a more conservative role for a woman doctor because she related Chinese recognition of her successes in what many readers doubtlessly recognized as a womanly approach to public health.

Gale reported that her expertise in public health was held in as high regard by the Chinese as her surgical skills. Chief of Police Yien recalled: "A year ago I opened a department for vaccination for the city with Dr. Gale's valuable help . . . no small-pox has ever occurred. In order to show a part of my personal appreciation for Dr. Gale's hard and assiduous work. . . . I formally reported the case to our central government through our Civil Governor Tsi." Chief of Police Yien received a command from the Ministry of Home Affairs at Peking acknowledging what he described as Gale's extreme concern for the public good. In recognition of Gale, Civil Governor Tsi prepared a merit board (a large banner to be paraded through the streets and posted on a wall) praising Gale. Civil Governor Tsi compared Gale to an ancient physician named Dr. Dung, who treated patients without monetary compensation, and instead planted one almond tree for each free treatment given a patient.[17]

Governor Tsi had likened Gale's medical work to Dung's almond forest, and in so doing, compared her to a gentleman and scholar held in high esteem by Chinese society. Dung was the classical Confucian doctor, planting almond trees for the good of the public, performing his duties as an avocation, out of purely humanitarian and philanthropic motives. The Chinese respected him as a member of the literati, the highest class. While Chinese tradition had classified surgical duties as "manual labor" (of low status), Governor Tsi had departed from this view in his assessment of Gale as both a good surgeon and a good public health physician.[18]

Gale's surgical and public health work was primarily motivated by a desire to serve the Lord, rather than for monetary gain. Thus, one can see a relationship between traditional Chinese society's esteem for philanthropically motivated medicine and Chinese appreciation for the work of Gale and other women medical missionaries motivated by piety and its nonmonetary rewards.

Chinese recognition was especially important for supporters' perceptions of Gale during the post–World War I period, as mainstream American culture manifested a decline in enthusiasm for the broad based, environmental approach to public health and opted instead for a laboratory-based, scientific approach. While public health became professionalized during the Progressive era, its leaders were men, and the field's emphases changed. As one historian noted, "the approach of locating, identifying and isolating bacteria and their human costs" was perceived as "a more elegant and efficient way of dealing with disease."[19] Thus, the Progressive era introduced a new hero, the medical scientist: the physician who valued "technical expertise" over the humanistic medicine embodied in earlier forms of public health work. Importantly, the discourse of both types of public health work were gendered. The scientific approach reflected values associated with men: rationality, objectivity and belief in the importance of isolating the bacteria, rather than treating the patient's overall health. As Regina Markell Morantz-Sanchez has noted, "the passing of progressivism deprived women physicians of a particular kind of social validation."[20]

Conversely, Gale reported not only social, but official validation for her efforts in China. This validation was likely experienced by women supporters when they read Gale's quarterly mission field letters, and when the contents of those letters reached the secular press, as was the case in 1919, when the *San Francisco Examiner* printed the proclamation of Nanchang's Chief of Police. The caption read: "Chinese Honor Bay City Woman: Public Recognition Accorded work of Dr. Ailie S. Gale of Oakland by Official."[21]

Gale's and other twentieth-century women missionaries' apparent successes in China were in part owed to the persistence of Confucianist medical ethics.[22] The value placed on "humaneness" (jen) and "compassion" (tz'u) was as evident in twentieth-century China as it had been five decades earlier, when Li Hung-chang provided support for Dr. Leonora Howard's medical work for women and children in Tientsin. While as a "cultural imperialist," Gale sought to impose her conception of medicine, she did so in a manner which complemented, rather than displaced, entrenched Confucian medical ethics. Moreover, supporters learned from Gale that Chief of Police Yien had been the one to organize the vaccination clinic and that she had helped him rather than directed him.

It is likely that Gale took direction from the chief of police because she held a degree of respect for the Chinese. This respect was evidenced during the post–World War I period when the Methodist Board gave Gale the opportunity to plan the reconstruction of the Nanchang General Hospital. When the Methodist Board worked in conjunction with the Rockefeller Foundation to initiate the project of rebuilding the Nanchang General Hospital, beginning in 1915, Gale soon found herself in charge of selecting the appropriate plans for the reconstruction project.[23] The opportunity to provide input into the selection of blue prints for the new design of the hospital let Gale articulate her views regarding the role of China medical missions. These views are important because they would later become an aspect of Gale's writings to supporters, and, in part, they help one understand Gale's attitude toward the Chinese.

In August 1920, Gale corresponded with Dr. J. G. Vaughan, who was in New York City handling the fund-raising aspects of the construction project. Gale reported that she had been gathering information from professionals, looking at the plans of other hospitals, and soliciting opinions from all Nanchang missionaries for over one year. She cited the unanimous agreement of all missionaries that the site was ample enough to build a hospital as large as some of the best hospitals in the United States and that the work should begin.

Vaughan's assignment was to secure more land for the hospital site. Perhaps because of his assigned duty, he believed that much more time and land was needed in order to have a site large enough for the hospital buildings.[24]

Gale had supported her position to Vaughan by citing the opinion of reputable individuals, including the entire community of missionaries. Several months later, however, in a letter to the new incoming Dr. Blydenburgh, Gale revealed that her urgency stemmed not so much from the certainty that the entire community supported this view, but from her awareness of the needs of the Chinese medical staff with whom she worked. Gale described her assistant Dr. Lee's persistent requests for an adequate physicians' residence far enough away from the hospital to provide a distinct line between the home and work area. Gale reiterated Lee's daily frustration with having to eat his meals directly above the kitchen, where the nurses dined. On one occasion, Lee had grown so annoyed at having to eat at the hospital, and anxious at the nurses' presence and chatter that he moved their tables to the front door of the hospital operating room.[25]

Gale's belief in the necessity that the Chinese medical staff be adequately housed led her to conclude that the most pressing need of the construction project was the building of a physicians' residence on the old site of Dr. Vaughan's house, a distance away from the hospital. Vaughan objected that Gale's site for the Chinese physicians' residence was inappropriate precisely due to its distance from the hospital. Concerned with his ability to manage Chinese physicians, and aware of Gale's emphasis on Chinese wishes for a separation from their work environment, Vaughan's retort was a powerful one:

> It may be that my thought of the term "future hospital development" has had a little different meaning than your own thought of the future hospital development. . . . I would put this hospital compound in a separate place by itself. I would run a thick wall, low perhaps and . . . with vines, down through the compound and then I would include in this hospital compound area a small compound space for the Chinese physicians' houses. It might be in the future that we would also have to put a Chinese pastors' residence in here. I am quite definitely convinced that we can not satisfactorily administer our medical work without having our Chinese physicians nearer to the site than any other available place would put them.[26]

Gale's view of the term "future hospital development" was supported by her husband. Reverend Francis Gale was enthusiastically and consistently involved in his wife's medical work, and he did not fall short of expressing this to his superiors. In his 1921 Nanchang Conference Budget report to the Methodist Board, he showed strong support of his wife's opinion. He too brought attention to the urgency of building a physicians' residence, noting that the hospital:

> shall never be able to keep a native physician content to remain here so long as he and his family are compelled to live in the present quarters over the hospital kitchen. It should not continue so another month. We ask that funds for the hospital be released.[27]

While Gale believed in the necessity of supervising the work of the Chinese, she appeared to place a higher priority on their needs. Gale's emphases may have stemmed from her experience training male nurses for the Nanchang General Hospital and female nurses for Dr. Ida Kahn's Hospital. She had expressed admiration for her Chinese nurses, remarking upon their hard work and competence, while admitting to supporters that several had not been Christians.[28] In short, for Vaughan, the priority was the mission's need to both acquire land and to assure maximum control over administration of the medical work. Gale worked closely with Chinese medical professionals, and her priority was to give them the work environment they believed they needed, regardless of whether the individuals had accepted Western religious beliefs.

Gale placed special emphasis upon the needs of Chinese women. While her hospital served both genders, during Vaughan's absence, Gale had worked to increase the number of female patients, bringing their percentage to one-third of inpatients. Having done so, Gale informed Vaughan that her specifications to the Board reflected their increasing numbers. Gale had set aside 34 of the 135 beds for women, and provided for a surgical ward of 11 beds, an obstetrical ward with 6 beds, a delivery room and a nursery. In addition, to accommodate women of different economic circumstances, there were 2 private rooms with a bath and 4 without.[29]

When one compares Gale's emphasis on meeting Chinese needs with Vaughan's stress on land acquisition and facile hospital administration, a possible conclusion is that the desire for power was not as significant a motivation for her as for him. However, Gale's request for 135 beds had been motivated by a sense of competition: she knew that the French Catholics were building a hospital nearby with 200 beds.[30]

While Gale's concern with keeping up with the French Catholics reflected a desire for dominance, she and Vaughan had exhibited a difference in perspective. Gale had suggested that the mission offer as much as other competitors so that Methodism, or Western Protestantism could retain influence among the Chinese. Vaughan, who had sought power through larger land acquisition, supported only an 80 bed hospital.[31] Vaughan had questioned whether the Methodist Board would ever be able to raise the funds for such a high number of beds and had not offered to help in petitioning to attain the additional funds necessary for them.[32] In short, Gale's behavior reflected the desire to dominate and influence through the typically female affinity for meeting the needs of Chinese patients and fellow doctors.

Gale's emphasis upon the needs of the Chinese, and the privileged status Gale enjoyed as the recipient of monies from the home field, served to reinforce her status as a representative of an imperialist power. Gale sent yearly Nanchang Hospital reports and included additional letters to all those who were especially interested in the hospital work.[33] In these letters, the success of the women's monies was tied to the power accorded Gale. While the Board did not formally recognize her as the chief administrator of the Nanchang Hospital, her letters implied that she was. When women of the Simpson Church wrote to Gale they discussed "your hospital," and she acknowledged that, for all intents and purposes, it was indeed hers. Gale established a connection between the women's support and her power within the hospital.[34] Reciprocity was established between Gale, in charge of the hospital, and supporters, whose gifts and monies for the family salary had contributed to her leadership position.

When Gale provided supporters with consistent, detailed information regarding her medical work, assuring them that their money had borne fruit, she also reinforced notions of supporters' privileged status vis-a-vis their Chinese beneficiaries. Gale provided supporters with specific recognition of their contributions to her work among the Chinese people, giving detailed accounts of each gift received. Gale described the exact reaction of the recipients, both missionary and Chinese, carefully noting the gift's utilization, while consistently reiterating heart-felt thanks. For example, Gale described how the "little baby carriages went to delight the heart of the little daughter of my bible woman." She often thanked the individual donors by name and promised one woman "who sent the doll" that she would receive a picture of the little girl to whom it went.[35]

The broad scope of Gale's correspondence indicates that her goal was not simply to fulfill the minimal Methodist Board requirements for quarterly letters to Parish Abroad supporters. While Gale was not formally a WFMS missionary, she found the time to both request gifts for the Ida Kahn Hospital and send letters of appreciation to the WFMS and the various women's groups within the Simpson Church, such as those in the Queen Esther circle.[36] The Board was pleased with the content of her letters and expressed appreciation for Gale's ability to communicate her successes to supporters.[37]

Gale's first phase of work in Nanchang had afforded her an opportunity to express to contributors an example of what American women would consider a rare anomaly: Gale was a female doctor in charge of many phases of medical work in a city with a population of over one million. She was an administrator, asked by the male-administered Methodist Episcopal Board of Missions, for her specifications for the construction of a hospital as large as some of the best hospitals in America. In doing so, Gale had expressed her view of the future of missionary medicine in China, and had simultaneously portrayed an image of Chinese professionals that went beyond the simple idea of supervising their efforts.

As hospital administrator and surgeon, Gale neither intimidated readers as unwomanly, nor projected stable images of home and hearth. In part this was owed to the nature of Gale's marriage, reflection of Gale's self-representation as a modern woman. As evidenced by his support for Gale's views regarding the reconstruction of the Nanchang General Hospital, Francis Gale championed his wife's opinions and professional needs. In fact, according to their son Frank Gale's recollections, the joke around the mission compound was the frequency and constancy with which Francis Gale reiterated the talents of his wife. Observers noted that Ailie Gale was the decision-maker in the marriage, that she believed herself superior to her husband, and that he apparently accepted this. Francis Gale could not help but pepper his correspondence to the United States with references to his wife's expert surgical performances and successful treatment of officials. Immediately upon arrival to China, Francis Gale had not mentioned the difficulties encountered, but instead chose to note that his wife was "certainly a 'cracker-jack'; for there has not been a single case that she has not been successful with where there was any possibility for recovery."[38]

Despite the brief period from 1913 to 1915, when Dr. Gale was in the United States on furlough due to the ill health caused by the miscarriage of the Gales' fourth child, supporters were told that her role as a mother had not conflicted with the strides she had made in her medical work. The household salary of $2,100 per year was large enough to enable Gale to work as a doctor by day, leaving her house in the care of what she described to supporters as a very competent Chinese staff. The mission salary was, by American standards, below the poverty line; however, in China the Gales had a cook, a waiter, who took care of the living and dining rooms, halls and Reverend Gale's study, an amah, or nanny who took care of the children and the upstairs bedrooms and bathrooms, a handy man, who, along with the other servants, lived in the basement area, and a gardener. In the evenings Gale would return home from her extensive medical duties and give her children the rudiments of an elementary school education. Indeed, immediately upon arrival in 1909, Francis Gale noted that his wife "seems to me to look better every day. I am sure that not having to do any of the house work is giving her an opportunity to get rest." Significantly, he saw no contradiction between his observation that his wife was rested and that she was simultaneously "up to her neck in medical work."[39]

Gale's dual combination of traditional and modern womanhood was especially significant during the first and second decades of the twentieth century as the Chinese Republic manifested signs of emulating Western ways. Within the backdrop of optimism for the new republic, many types of American women, conservative and feminist, were given reason to possibly identify with Gale and find contentment in her self-representation. Like many women missionaries, Gale may have been perceived as a role model for the rapidly growing numbers of modernized Chinese women.

Women missionaries were particularly important in the post-1911 period, as missionaries began comparing the new Republican China, to the United States in its early Republican phase. Prior to the 1911 revolution, American missionaries had tended to emphasize the need to elevate both the Chinese nation and its women;[40] however, with the 1911 revolution the emphasis came increasingly to be on the similarity between both cultures. Yuan Shih-kai, warlord turned president, and later emperor, was heralded by missionaries as a legitimate leader and sometimes compared to early American leaders. Sun Yat-sen was compared to the American George Washington. The overthrow of the Ch'ing Dynasty and the subsequent warlord battles resulting from China's quest for unification were compared to the internal and foreign threats against the early American republic.[41] In April 1912, Gale reminded supporters that it would be "many years before China will be adjusted to her new form of government and until then there will be trouble." However, she asked that they recall "how long it took our own country to reach a settled condition."[42]

With the overthrow of the Ch'ing Dynasty and the emphasis upon Sino-American similarities, missionaries began to find affinities between the women of both nations.[43] Many Chinese women had begun their fight for a public role in the new democracy just as the women's suffrage movement reached its apogee in America. Many Chinese and Americans argued that their respective nations would benefit from granting women suffrage and a more public role because voting rights would allow women to use their ballots for the moral betterment of the nation.

Likewise, advances in the development of the Chinese Republic were correlated with advances for Chinese women. As one *China Christian Advocate* editorial expressed it, "If China is to be saved by its New Man . . . it must have the help of the new woman."[44]

When Nanchang missionary Welthy Honsinger observed that with the revolution there would be no more insignias of rank, she posited this alongside changes for Chinese women:

> The fire of devotion to the Republic burned high those days in the heart of every girl in China. . . . No one dares to prophesy the future of this country when her womanhood shall be unbound in body and mind and spirit.[45]

It is not surprising, given the confluence between Chinese national development, increasing public rights for women, and comparisons between China and the United States, that mission supporters would express their interest in the Chinese women their churches supported— women who came under the influence of women missionaries like Gale.[46]

In keeping with the post-1911 missionary tendency to depict Chinese women as paralleling American women in their struggles, Gale provided detailed descriptions of Chinese women's talents and other positive attributes. Supporters learned of upper-class ladies whom Gale treated for various ailments, then befriended and invited to dinner. For example, one was an artist, the other a capable administrator who directed an officially sponsored Nanchang exhibition in 1911. Clearly, the new Chinese woman was not one who remained restricted to the confines of her home, but was gifted and confident of her new role.[47]

With what was a standard cultural superiority among missionaries, Gale optimistically discussed her wish to free those women that she perceived as less fortunate for a life of activity. Supporters were told of her "rare experience unbinding the feet of ten girls" from Nanchang's Baldwin School. It was no easy task, dressing their tiny feet "night and morning," but when one thought of what it was "going to mean to the lives of these girls where they shall be able to get around as normal women," it certainly paid off, she wrote.[48]

Gale's varied duties enabled her to describe many types of Chinese women. In addition to her medical duties Gale taught industrial classes at the Baldwin School. One Bible class in America supported a poor, thirty-eight-year old Chinese Bible woman, an expert needlewoman. Gale explained that the bible woman was an artist and she assisted Gale in working out designs and patterns for the girls in the classes. Supporters were sent a picture of the industrial class and told that their yarn and needles were used to teach girls to make marketable goods that would render them self-sufficient.[49]

Readers learned the most about Gale's views on Chinese women from her descriptions of her adopted Chinese daughter. On a bitterly cold November evening in 1912, Gale had just completed a day's work and set out to go home when the hospital nurses came to report that a one-month-old baby girl had been left outside the gate of the Nanchang Hospital. Gale took her home and Gale's sons convinced her to adopt the baby and name her Mary. Soon supporters began contributing money and gifts and expressing interest in Mary's progress.

Most missionaries did not adopt Chinese babies, however, Gale's treatment of Mary was typical of those who did. Her aim was to make sure that Mary was raised to appreciate her culture, learn the Chinese language and dress like a Chinese woman.[50] While Gale raised Mary as a Christian, she sent her to both government and Christian schools (the nearby Baldwin school in 1918). Gale aimed to instill a sense of national pride in Mary: "We have tried to impress upon her that she is Chinese and that she must plan her life so as to be of the most use to her own people."[51] With these goals in mind, Mary was trained from childhood for a career, a life of public service within the medical profession.

Mary's training had been in keeping with the general missionary atmosphere of optimism concerning Chinese women in the professions. A 1914 article in the *China Christian Advocate* had noted American Minister Paul Reinsch's awe during a commencement at North China Union Medical College for Women: China was so full of "new developments . . .

but nothing is so significant and so full of interest as the development of the medical science . . . profession . . . when two Chinese ladies are going to join the medical profession."[52] Two years later, the *China Christian Advocate* noted the "considerable number of lady doctors" who were members of the Chinese Medical Association, an organization of Western educated Chinese men and women. Could women readers help but compare this milestone in China to American women physicians' exclusion from participation in the American Medical Association?[53]

Gale's optimism for the new Chinese Republic included an observation of official approval for Chinese women in medicine. Like other women missionaries, Gale was aware of the power of Chinese women doctors as role models.[54] She noted that during the excitement of late 1911, the Governor of Nanchang, "the highest gentry man, together with the wives and families of a number of officials, rushed to Dr. Kahn's hospital to seek protection." Gale explained that the upper class Chinese had gone to Kahn's Hospital because "they had so much confidence in her and knew so well that the soldiers and officials would respect and protect her." During the excitement of the revolution, Nanchang residents had all left the city, but for weeks, Dr. Kahn's hospital was crowded.[55]

When the excitement had died down and conditions were settled, Gale noted Sun Yat-sen's visit to Nanchang and the new regime's significance to Christians and Chinese women:

> All the streets are gay with the new Chinese colors and all the soldiers are in their best uniforms. Groups are here and there along the bank of the river with canons every few hundred yards. The Governor has accepted for him an invitation to meet the Christians at Dr. Kahn's.[56]

Dr. Sun's speech on the following Sunday was warmly met, as was a subsequent speech from a Christian Chinese Yale graduate. When the speech was over, the audience and speakers all went to Dr. Kahn's for a celebration. Clearly, Gale perceived these as auspicious signs that Christianity would triumph with the victory of Republican leaders. Shortly afterward, Gale reported that three Buddhist nuns approached Dr. Kahn with a request for training as Bible women, offering their temple for a Christian Day School. Gale reported Kahn's observation that the Bible women had been part of a class of women "for a long time unreached" by the Christian message.[57]

American supporters gave evidence of interest in the overall progress made by Chinese women and were willing to provide financial support upon learning of Gale's impending work with them. During the early 1920s, the Board came to the decision of sending the Gales to Tunki, a remote region in the province of Anhwei. Ironically, while Gale was still not officially an appointed missionary and she was not receiving a salary, Bishop Birney was "counting" on her being "the woman who will win the hearts of the women." Despite Birney's vote of confidence, Gale felt that she needed to update her medical knowledge, especially in the field of surgery. She hoped to study while on furlough in the United States beginning in 1922.

The initial petition to the Board for the funding of Gale's courses was accompanied by Reverend Francis Gale's request for study of institutional church work. However, when the Board's reply was to point to the distressing deficit in its finances, Francis Gale dropped his own plea, reminding them of Gale's "devotion to the Nanchang Hospital," where she bore "burdens there greater than her physical strength warranted" with "not one penny of remuneration from the Board." Francis Gale's admonitions did not convince the Board, but friends from the Simpson Church agreed to contribute toward Gale's expenses. Thus, it was only with the help of supporters that Gale was able to take postgraduate medical courses at Columbia Medical College, and prepare for the new mission field in Tunki Anhwei.[58]

5

Chinese Nationalism and Public
Health Work in Tunki, Anhwei

GALE'S ABILITY TO SUSTAIN A STRONG BOND WITH CONTRIBUTORS
was tested most rigorously in the Tunki mission field, in the Wannan
District of Anhwei, from 1923–27. During this critical period, when
Methodist Board finances reached a nadir and Chinese Nationalists
threatened to dismantle Christian institutions, Gale would build what
she described as a small but thriving hospital with no Board funding.
Gale's work was financed exclusively by American mission field and local
Chinese supporters.[1] This chapter will describe how Gale cultivated
bonds between herself, friends in America and the Chinese, amidst the
uncertainties of a growing antiforeignism; and how these bonds let her
raise the funds needed to run her hospital and implement her medical
projects.

Methodist mission work in the Tunki area began in 1915 when Los Angeles businessman Milton Stewart donated three million dollars toward
Presbyterian and Methodist mission work in India and China. Stewart
stipulated that the money be used "to fill up what is lacking on the
evangelistic side of the mission work." In Tunki, part of the Stewart Fund
was used to support education and evangelistic work.[2] Dr. Milton Charles
had begun the medical work in Tunki in 1915. In the early 1920s, the
Board asked the Gales to take over the Tunki field: Reverend Gale could
continue the evangelical work and his wife could take over the medical
work from Dr. Charles, who was due for a furlough. In 1923 the Gales
arrived in Tunki with their fourteen-year-old son Frank and three male
nurses who had been trained by Gale in Nanchang.[3]

Gale expressed disappointment with conditions in Tunki, but she
did not communicate this disillusion to supporters. Shortly after their
arrival, the other two missionary couples, Dr. Charles and his wife and
Reverend and Mrs. Martin took their furloughs, leaving the Gales alone
on the field with newly converted Chinese Christians.[4] Gale described

what she defined as "spiritual weakness" on the part of the Chinese Christians on the field: The pastor's wife was having an extramarital affair, and her husband and two of the male teachers in the day school were selling "dope." Gale told the board that she and her husband responded to the existing situation by "clearing out all the offending" persons.[5]

According to Gale, their strongest weapon on the Tunki field during this difficult period was the medical work, which received no funding from the Board, but was the focus of Gale's letters.[6] Gale explained to the Board that readers did not need to know the negative aspects of mission work, and that sometimes "it is more help to the work to withhold information rather than give it." Astutely, she focused instead upon her greatest triumph: peoples' growing awareness that when they were "sick and in need of something," they could rely on her hospital.[7] Thus, while Gale had privately emphasized rigid moral codes and expressed intolerance for those whom she deemed "sinners," she subsumed this concern, understanding that readers primarily wanted information about her medical work.

While Gale's relationship with supporters followed the same lines established in Nanchang, there was a new intensity to the medical situation in Tunki. In Nanchang, a hospital, supported by Board appropriations, had been in existence when Gale arrived. In Tunki, Gale relied solely upon money and gifts from friends in the homeland for turning a house into a hospital.[8]

Gale's letters emphasized supporters' vital role in helping her create a hospital where none had existed. Upon arrival, Gale told supporters that their monies had covered the cost of renovating the house and paying one of her Nanchang nurses, Mr. Li to remain in the building to oversee the workmen.[9] Gale frequently provided lists of items needed, placing at least one advertisement in the *California Advocate* in 1924.[10] Supporters responded by selecting an item(s) from her list and obtaining a bank draft for its cost. Gale's letters to friends explained:

> The quickest way to send money is to get a draft from *your own* bank. Just tell them you want to send so much to China and they will write you out a draft which you inclose in your letter. When it comes, I send it to our treasurer and he exchanges it. In about 2 weeks after the letter arrives, the money can be used . . .[11]

In response to her circular letters, Gale received bank drafts from a variety of locations. Gale's 1923–24 hospital report indicated that the Simpson Church contributed the most, that year with $510.00. However, smaller amounts ranging from $100 to $5.00 came from individuals or organizations in Oakland, Pasadena, Coteti, and Petaluma, California, the hometown of Reverend Francis Gale, and Evanston, Illinois and Portland Oregon.[12]

While funds sent for the purchase of specific items reflected supporters' increasing awareness of the nature of Gale's hospital work, the gifts shipped from the United States revealed an even more personal connection. Such essentials as a hospital operating table and eye instruments had not been part of the medical work inherited by Gale from Dr. Charles. Gale requested these essentials immediately upon arrival, and by December 1924, one year later, the Simpson Church had already purchased them.[13] Smaller, less costly articles such as gauze bandages, yards of cotton fabric and muslin, pillow cases, aprons, clothes, pins, hooks, wash cloths, absorbing cotton, kitchen utensils, spools of adhesive plaster, pounds of antiseptic cotton, operating gowns and towels, came more frequently, intensifying each supporters' bond with Gale's work.

New and used clothing, blankets, books, Victrola records, shoes and dolls, would be donated to Chinese Christians. All of these served as a link between supporters and everyday mission life in China.[14] Items were secured through a vast communications network which baffled even Gale. In one instance, Gale received valuable hospital goods from four New York churches "of which we had never heard," because someone unknown to her had placed an advertisement in a *New York Advocate* on her behalf.[15] Gale reminded supporters that these small, frequent gifts meant less expenses for the hospital and more free and low-cost treatment for the Chinese.[16]

While in Nanchang, Gale had described how American gifts were utilized by recipients, but during her years in Tunki, Gale was more detailed and emphatic in her descriptions. In exchange for their contributions, supporters were given the impression that their influence over the Chinese was even greater than in the past. She linked American gifts to patients' good feelings about both Gale's medical expertise and Christianity.

For example, she told of one eleven-year-old boy who had blown holes through both legs while playing with a Chinese gun. While he had arrived at the hospital weak from the loss of blood and Gale feared that he might die on the operating table, she treated him successfully and he improved. Gale informed Miss Burtis, of the Simpson Church, that her father's jacket had covered the boy's entire body for one month as his bloodied clothes, the only thing he owned, had become useless. Gale described how the "brightest little fellow" she had ever seen was so grateful for his treatment that he will be coming to "our day school next year."[17]

For many months, a man with cataracts had come every day to inquire about the eye instruments that Gale had ordered from the United States. Finally, in April 1925, Gale told supporters that she had received the instruments while in the midst of a busy morning of surgical work, and was preparing to remove the man's cataracts.[18]

Acknowledgment of supporters' generosity was coupled with Gale's descriptions of Chinese gratitude and apparent confidence in her work: she had been told that "people would be afraid of us, but only a few have been. The majority have seemed real friendly." Gale told supporters that this friendliness and confidence resulted in significant financial support for Gale's hospital.[19]

Gale wrote that since the clinic opened in April 1924, "we have treated more than a hundred" patients per week, therefore, the "prospects are encouraging." The hospital would formally open on 2 June 1924.[20] Hospital reports submitted by Gale to the Board and supporters indicated a steady increase in confidence among Chinese patients. The hospital had treated 2,216 male and 440 female outpatients from 1923–24, and the numbers for 1924–25 were 4,120 and 1,085, respectively. The wealthier patients had provided Gale's hospital with $748.30 from 1924-25, enabling her to give 276 free treatments to the poor. Indeed, from 1924–25, local contributions from the Chinese totaled $1,741.99, surpassing the $1,467.49 received from America.[21]

Gale's hospital reports not only emphasized Chinese support, but also Gale's expertise as an administrator. She had started 1924 with a surplus of $38.43 and finished with a balance of $720.00. She used her surplus on medical supplies essential for the hospital's continued growth, establishing a fund for various items such as a microscope, more instruments, and drugs.[22]

Gale's expertise in raising money from both American and Chinese sources contrasted starkly with the bleak financial condition of Methodist Episcopal Church Board during the 1920s. While women's groups in American churches (the WFMS, the Queen Esther Girls, and the Ladies Aid Societies) had continued to maintain a high level of enthusiasm toward women professionals abroad, men had begun to lose interest in missions.

This waning interest in missions stemmed from a general post–World War I disillusionment, exacerbated by the problems faced within Protestant churches. In the past, pastors had had the time to exhort their congregations through meetings, prayer days, and other special events; however, in the 1920s, poorly paid pastors with mounting responsibilities rarely devoted energy to the missionary cause. The resultant decrease in total mission funds collected through the World Service Commission forced the Methodist Board to consider closing certain missionary fields by the 1920s.[23]

Despite Gale's assertions of financial and professional astuteness and the support of her medical work among women, the Board threatened to close the newly established Tunki mission, reasoning that the newest fields should be the first to close. While World Service appropriations may not have been needed for Gale's medical work, evangelical and educational work in Tunki depended upon appropriations from the rapidly diminishing Stewart Fund.

Gale's response to the Board was echoed in letters to supporters. She pointed out that the Tunki field might be new but it was more successful than many of the older mission fields. Proof of this lay in Tunki citizens' loyalty toward the mission and its medical work during a precarious time for China mission work.[24]

Gale's letters to supporters were written amidst the backdrop of the rising Chinese nationalism of the 1920s, and her accounts of success in Tunki can best be understood in light of the virulent anti-Christian feeling gripping China at this time. The movement was an outgrowth of circumstances originating in 1898, 1911 and the First World War.

Missionaries had expressed much optimism for the new Chinese Republic in the years after 1911; however, Yuan Shih-kai's attempt at empire and his subsequent death had been followed by a civil war between competing power holders in a disunified China. Tension heightened as the forces of capitalism and imperialism came to a head in World War I. The war had brought burgeoning industry and a rising new Chinese merchant class. In Shanghai, Tientsin, and Wuhan, towns and industrial centers developed and the treaty port merchant class grew accordingly; however, this class had imbibed Western nationalism along with capitalism, and before long many nationalistic Chinese, and the former beneficiaries of Western protection came to protest the presence of foreign-made goods in China.

During World War I, China also experienced aggressive Japanese imperialism, resulting in the eventual political, economic and territorial concessions that were the Japanese government's "Twenty-one Demands." The post-1918 period brought disappointment for nationalistic Chinese, as wartime assurances of Wilsonian support against Japan gave way to the Chinese betrayal at the Versailles Peace Conference, where Japan was permitted to maintain control over the former German concessions in Shantung, in exchange for cooperation for Wilson's League of Nations.[25]

China's May Fourth Movement, begun in 1919, embodied both merchant class anger and a more intellectually based Nationalist indignation at Japanese encroachment. With China's signing of the Treaty of Versailles, merchants' dissatisfaction converged with the discontent that had been brewing in Chinese universities since the late nineteenth century.

Student protests during the May Fourth Movement were the climax to a series of serious letdowns for Chinese intellectuals: they had been unfulfilled by the constitutional reform movement of 1898 and the revolution of 1911. By 1919, the feeling of national humiliation and urgency caused by events at Versailles translated into a strong impetus for action. Students centered at Peking University planned a mass demonstration for 7 May, the National Day of Humiliation, but tensions erupted early, and on 4 May they protested against the Peking government leaders who had sold out China for personal gain. The mass demonstration became a strike, as students filled the streets, distributing leaflets and making speeches. Their power was magnified when they were joined by nationalistic merchants who closed their shops in support of the students.

Anti-imperialist protests continued into 1920. Labor unions (organized among the large factory labor class that had developed during World War I) joined merchants and students in a broad demonstration of national feeling in China.[26]

The 1920s saw the forces of protest that had gained momentum in post World War I coalesce into an even greater anti-imperialist, anti-Christian, action-oriented platform. Christianity was attacked on several fronts: intellectuals like Dr. Hu Shih, a pragmatist, pointed out Christianity's conflict with science. Merchants and labor classes singled out missionaries as representatives of Western domination and as "running dogs of imperialism."

The preeminent Nationalist leader among intellectuals was the missionary-educated Sun Yat-sen, who sought to complete a revolution based upon the idea of mass movements and anti-imperialism. Sun's Nationalist, or Kuomintang party had cooperated with the Soviet Union in the hopes of broadening the base of the Chinese revolution, beginning in 1923.[27] The anti-imperialism and patriotism of the Kuomintang was reflected in the events beginning in late 1924 and climaxing with the 30 May Incident of 1925.

In this milieu, beginning in December 1924, student strikes caused almost complete anarchy in missionary schools in Central and Southern China, particularly in the province of Hunan. A number of political leaders and Kuomintang party officials in Canton supported more protest as the months progressed.[28] Then on 30 May 1925, Shanghai students and laborers joined together in a momentous protest.

Workers at Japanese textile mills had been on strike since December 1924. Violent riots had resulted in the death of a striker on 15 May, and on

30 May, students and laborers entered the International Settlement with anti-Japanese banners. British officers attempted to push back the crowd; however, angry protesters pushed forward, demanding justice for murdered Chinese and cancellation of the unequal treaties. A British officer shot at the crowd of protesters, wounding seventeen and killing twelve. The Shanghai Incident, referred to as the "Boston Tea Party" of the Chinese revolution, set China aflame with more strikes, boycotts and riots.[29]

When news of Chinese antiforeignism reached American supporters, many wrote to the Gales expressing concern for their safety.[30] However, throughout the family's stay in Tunki, Gale consistently emphasized that the hospital was untouched by the anti-Christian sentiments prevailing throughout most Tunki and all of China. Throughout the two-year period, from 1925 to 1927, Gale attained a great deal of credibility among supporters by attributing most of her successes with Tunki residents to both her own doing and that of talented Chinese Christians.

There were three government schools near the Gales, one for women and two for boys, with a total enrollment of about one thousand students. Students there had covered the city with anti-British and anti-Japanese placards and endeavored to raise funds for Shanghai strikers. Gale assured supporters that student protests did not reach the hospital because it was run by friendly Americans rather than hostile British or Japanese subjects. Gale credited herself and her hospital as a factor in Tunki residents' lack of animosity toward her.

Upon arrival to Tunki in 1923, Gale had hired three male graduates of one of the nearby government schools as students of nursing. Soon she befriended the Buddhist teachers and pupils of that school. This friendship had not prevented the school from sympathizing with strikers, but it had prevented them from undertaking anti-Christian activities against the hospital.[31]

Gale's choice of employees had had another important affect: the hospital was not targeted by Chinese Nationalist sentiment, but rather was given military protection. One of the three Buddhist nurses initially hired by Gale was the son of a colonel who had charge of the squad of soldiers stationed in Tunki. This squad marched around the foot of the hill surrounding the hospital, protecting it each evening.[32] For Gale, the hospital's need for protection took precedence over the necessity to understand the motivations for Chinese protest. In fact, during these years, Gale was opposed to Chinese protests of any kind. The beginning of 1925 had seen not only increasing Chinese nationalism but also the start of Gale's public health campaign. Letters to supporters juxtaposed the success of this medical campaign with the message that the anti-Christian movement had still not touched the Tunki Hospital.[33]

She viewed any antiforeign activity as a threat which would be fore-stalled by the success of her medical endeavors. Apparently indifferent to Japanese imperialism's real threat to China, Gale showed no sympathy for Chinese protests. Focused singularly on her own goals, Gale noted that when Christianity and public health flourished, anti-Japanese feeling dissipated: she described to supporters that while government school students were busy distributing "kill the Japs" pamphlets, her nurses were busy going around the shops distributing literature entitled, "kill the fly," which she considered a more reasonable message.[34]

In July 1925, her Tunki nurses suggested the idea of sending three hundred booklets on "kill the fly" and one hundred booklets on "foot-binding" to the large government school (Buddhist) from which they had graduated in 1924. Supporters were told of the nurses' request and the letter of appreciation they received from the school's devout Buddhist principal.[35]

Gale noted that American magazines informed supporters that China's students had vowed to make as much trouble as possible for Christians between 25 and 28 December 1925, so she presented her medical expertise as an essential force deflecting this trouble. For example, in the fall of 1925, Gale paid a house-visit to one of Tunki's wealthiest families, where an elderly woman, an opium smoker, had been so close to death that a photographer had come to take the traditional final snap-shot. While given little detail, supporters were told that Gale easily cured the terrified woman. The woman's son, who was not a Christian, informed Gale that he would be sending a Merit Board and asked if she wanted it presented at the hospital or clinic. Eager to flaunt her success, Gale decided upon the clinic, reasoning that because people passed through there from morning until night, it would make more of an impact upon the Tunki populace.

On the "auspicious" day of 28 December, a five-foot-long, flamingo red enameled Merit Board arrived with four big gold-painted characters stating: "The gospel that is beneficial to the Age." The twelve carriers holding the message were accompanied by eighty students from three private schools and twenty musicians. For the duration of the Gales' time in Tunki, the Merit Board hung permanently above the clinic entrance.[36]

It was the lack of antiforeignism on the part of Tunki Chinese, Christians and non-Christians, which led to the Board's decision, in the summer of 1925, to maintain the Gales in the field, at least for the time being. Gale reported to friends in the homeland that "The enthusiasm of the Chinese brethren was an inspiration." They proposed to supervise their own work, an idea that Gale claimed to have supported all along. When the new Chinese pastor and district superintendent arrived, Gale deemed them the "most spiritual men" of the Central China conference.[37]

Despite the backdrop of an anti-Christian China, Gale had depicted herself as able to use her medical and social skills to deflect hostility and inspire confidence among Tunki residents. Gale apparently convinced supporters enough to inspire continued contributions. Gale's show of support for Chinese professionals encouraged even further American mission field contributions. On 18 November 1925, Gale asked the home field for $1,000 in order to expand the building structure of her hospital, or as she put it, "raise the roof."[38]

As in Nanchang, Gale emphasized that an important priority was the needs of Chinese professionals: she explained that the nurses were crowded in one building and needed more comfortable quarters. Secondly, if nurses were given additional space, more hospital space would then be available for patients. Ninety-two people had been willing to show their faith by staying for treatment "but could not because there was an insufficient number of beds for in-patients."[39]

Gale's request was made at a time when the Methodist Board's financial state continued to be bleak. On 30 December 1925, she told the Simpson Church that she would again have no assistance from the Methodist Board. However, she declared herself undisturbed at the prospect of having to carry the hospital "without any money from regular appropriations" because

> So many friends put a little gift in their letters and since we returned a month ago $112 [gold] has come that way. Everyone seems so interested. It seems almost weird the way those letters go—friend sends on to friends in other parts of the country. A gift has just come in from a Congregational church where they receive the letters.[40]

Less than four months later, Gale reported receiving $853.00 and two weeks after that, $300 each from one friend in Southern California and from the Simpson Church, giving her well over the $1,000 requested.[41] Throughout 1926 and 1927, Gale's letters to supporters continued to inspire steady gifts of goods and monies from America, most of which came directly to her rather than through the New York office of the Methodist Episcopal Board of Foreign Missions.[42]

Gale's success at inspiring supporters' contributions had been owed to her self-representation as a competent physician. Importantly, it was also linked to her assurances of Chinese faith in her public health campaign.

Gale's one-year-old public health campaign reached its zenith of popularity among Tunki residents and officials in May 1926, while Kuomintang armies planned their year long march to unify China.[43] While Nationalist revolutionary armies successfully made their way from Canton to the Yangtze valley to drive out the Peking Government in the Northern Expedition of 1926–27, supporters read Gale's account of another battle won: on behalf of preventative medicine, and against the mosquito.

In Tunki, where more people succumbed to malaria than any other disease, Gale reported to supporters that her public health campaigns had finally borne fruit. As she explained in May 1926, the culmination of her efforts was a one-week campaign on public health, the result of which was a "real hit." During the campaign, school children marched in health parades, nurses and religious workers carried banners and Chinese national flags, musicians entertained and nurses gave health lectures on city sanitation.

Within the week, Gale reported success. New wire screens covered over dozens of fruit and candy shops, a vendor peddled securely protected candy, a school teacher told children "to buy candy only from sellers who thus protected their sweets," and four shops developed a land office business in the manufacturing of screens. One man, a manufacturer, was distributing handbills for screen covers and wind-cupboards to every Tunki shop. For emphasis, Gale enclosed a copy of the handbill in her letter to supporters.[44]

From the American perspective, Gale's work doubtlessly appeared exciting in light of the extensive research being conducted on the practical control of infectious diseases such as malaria and hook worm.[45] Within the parameters of medical missionary work in the 1920s, Gale's public health campaign had even broader ramifications. As Regina Markell Morantz-Sanchez notes, "In the 1920s women physicians remained strongly identified with public health at a time when the glitter of a public health career began to fade."[46] In China, as in the United States, it was never a part of the mainstream of medical missionary work. One 1925 survey of 210 missionary hospitals (out of a total of about 326) indicated that 84.8 percent declared hospital/dispensary work to be of primary importance and only 53.5 percent placed public health work second in importance.[47]

While Gale's was a self-directed and self-administered campaign, men played a very large part in its success. On a personal level, Gale told supporters that she could have done nothing without the help of her husband Francis Gale, her "right-hand man."[48] Likewise, Gale insisted that her knowledgeable male nurses seemed to have unending enthusiasm for public health: she reported that they were relentless in handing out literature and giving lectures on hygiene.

Importantly, Chinese men were very receptive to Gale's ideas. Each evening of her campaign, a different symbol of Chinese male authority agreed to attend: on Tuesday evening the police force and on Wednesday, members of the Chamber of Commerce, one of whom suggested usage of the large Tunki tea factories as lecture areas in the next demonstration. The Chief of Police, (a boyhood friend of the Chinese pastor, Mr. Shen) regularly supervised the sweeping of streets for the first time in Tunki's history. The Chief of Police also helped with the suppression of opium and gambling, and he had attended and supported Gale's one-week campaign. American supporters were informed that on one evening, soldiers brought their bugles and drums, paraded the area and attended the health lectures at the Methodist Church. Gale's readers were told that news of the soldiers' attendance "soon spread" to other areas, thus providing further validation for Gale.[49]

Gale's apparent success with soldiers in the area of public health was reflective of a larger phenomenon: her hospital's apparent ability to neutralize these fighting men, rendering them innocuous. Southern soldiers had arrived in Kiangsi and engaged in a bloody battle by September of 1926. Northern soldiers who had been defeated in the Kiangsi campaign, reached Gale's Hospital by 18 November 1926. In her correspondence, Gale showed preference for neither the Northern nor Nationalist cause, emphasizing only her ability to use Simpson Church funds to enhance her hospital's capacity to serve the men she depicted as victims of war.

Gale's letters offered a link between the wartime experiences of Chinese soldiers and the contributions of supporters to the Tunki Hospital. Gale expressed outrage as one Northern soldier related the fate of three thousand killed during the fighting near the city of Nanchang.[50] As the Nationalist campaign progressed, increasing numbers of wounded Northern soldiers made their way to the Tunki Hospital, causing a strain in hospital resources. The Simpson Church's gifts of muslin were made into sheets by Chinese girls who had taken refuge in Gale's home. The extra sheets enabled the hospital to take in more patients. Supporters' gifts of gauze, cotton and plaster disappeared by the pound, as the soldiers had to be "dressed daily." Importantly, monies set aside to "raise the roof" would be utilized sooner than expected: the presence of soldiers necessitated more expansion—an immediate action made possible by supporters' donations.[51]

When Americans expressed their worry over Northern soldiers' presence in the Tunki Hospital, Gale assured them that, despite the "terrible reputation" of the men, in her presence they had "behaved splendidly." Rather, the soldiers were a "grateful bunch" and Gale did not expect any trouble from them.[52] Gale's hospital, located on the hilltop was described as "the haven to which many turned for help," and Gale told supporters that the Chinese believed it was "the safest place in Tunki."[53] Gale's confidence in her hospital's safety continued even after she received word from the Bishop that "Southern troops, if they get in, will do some fierce stunts, as they have done in other places."[54]

While Gale told supporters about disturbing slogans advocated by the Nationalist Government, such as "Down with imperialism," and "Strike the Catholic and Protestant Churches," she did not interpret these as cause to doubt her presence in China. In March 1927, when Southern soldiers were "expected any day now," Gale had still believed it unnecessary to leave, reiterating her hospital's ability to mollify soldiers:

> The little hospital is a wonderful peace bringer. We still have four Northern soldiers in the hospital. They have parted with their uniforms and are now just patients which has relieved their anxiety greatly.[55]

Gale also believed that the support of Tunki officials was reason enough to stay. Tunki's military officials and soldiers, accompanied by the police commissioner and a squad of police, had paid a formal visit, presenting a Merit Board of the "finest" quality, and requesting that the Gales remain.[56]

When the American Consulate ordered an evacuation from Tunki in April 1927, Gale packed the family belongings unwillingly, naively continuing to believe that "there wasn't the least bit" of antiforeign feeling.[57] Soon, however, Gale began to view the situation with more realism. Describing her 1927 departure, Gale said: "It seemed needless for us, but when we saw the faces of our friends on arrival in Shanghai, we knew that things had been more serious than we had dreamed."[58]

The Gales arrived in Shanghai, joining over seventy-five thousand other foreigners and about three million Chinese who lived in the city on 10 April 1927. Soon Gale took a position as physician and preceptress at the Shanghai American School. Gale's sons Lester and Frank were both attending the school at this time, and Reverend Francis Gale served as temporary principal.[59] For five years, from 1928 to 1933, Gale was committed by contract to the school.[60] As the principal of the school, Elam J. Anderson, explained it, the Gales took positions at the school because it was close enough to Tunki to make it possible for the couple to visit their former mission station.[61]

While at the Shanghai American School, Gale fulfilled her obligations as physician and preceptress, overseeing the students in the girls' dormitory, she expressed nostalgia for the Tunki field.[62] Upon hearing of her new duties, Gale's reaction was one of bewilderment. She worried that she would not know how to relate to young American women. She took solace in the fact that these girls, at the very least, were not those American "flappers" for whom she had felt a potent revulsion.[63] Two

former Shanghai American School students, contacted for the purposes
of this study, recalled very little of Gale, but much about her "ebullient"
husband, whom the students nicknamed "Papa Frank." Gale was described by one S.A.S. alumni as very, very reserved and serious. Another
recalled only that she was "a busy, active lady, always taking care of
responsibilities."[64] According to her son Frank, Gale was reserved with
everyone except the "Chinese with and for whom she worked."[65] Clearly,
Gale's heart was in Tunki, the topic of all her letters to supporters during
the period.

Gale was not permitted to visit her hospital again because the Board
had deemed it too dangerous; however, through her husband's visits and
subsequent reports, she encouraged friends in the homeland to continue
sending gifts to the Tunki field. In order to accomplish this goal from 1927
to 1931, Gale's letters to supporters emphasized the talents of Chinese
Christians remaining in the field.

Gale's correspondence from Shanghai to the homeland emphasized
that despite her absence, evidence of her influence remained. Gale's
trained nurses had "been carrying on very well" since her departure
and they communicated regularly, sending reports of receipts from local
Chinese patients. A nurse named Li had been Gale's apprentice for ten
years, and he now did a "fine job" of seeing large numbers of patients
and managing the medical work. Gale's absence would not preclude
the continuance of her public health campaigns and its effect on the
Tunki populace was still strong: Reverend Gale reported that vendors
still covered their wares with glass and screens.[66]

An important symbol of the success of Chinese Christian efforts was
Mr. Shen, who was both pastor and district superintendent in Tunki.
Gale projected Shen as proof that the Tunki mission had been a success:
he was both highly principled and brave. Gale reported that the local
Kuomintang party in Tunki not only asked Shen to speak, but seemed
to acquiesce to his Christian teachings. At one meeting of two hundred
Nationalists, a local person made "a most violent address against imperialism." Gale reiterated her husband's account of Shen's masterful response
and its reflection of Chinese capabilities. Later, many of the guests praised
Shen for his courage. Gale predicted that Tunki's military, civil officials,
and businessmen would all come under Shen's influence. Shen's was not
a lone voice in the wilderness when it came to depicting the Nationalists
as amenable to Christian influence.

Francis Gale reported that after March 1927, when revolutionary
troops reached Nanking, attacking foreign residents and killing six, the
local magistrate of the hsien (county) proclaimed that anyone injuring
the Christian Church would be considered an enemy of the Nationalist

party.[67] In July 1927, three months after the Nanking Incident and Chiang's attack and decimation of Communist forces in Shanghai and Wuhan, Gale reported increased optimism among Tunki's Methodist preachers. In Tunki, Southern officers, officials, teachers, students, and businessmen had recently heard of Chiang's decree of protection for foreign property and were prompted to attend the Methodist Church one Sunday. While there, the new pastor preached on Sun Yat-sen's Three Principles and their relationship to the Christian Church. According to Shen, the crowd found the sermon gripping, and the reaction of Southern soldiers confirmed to him that the church would not be persecuted by Nationalists.[68] Clearly, correspondence indicates that as early as 1927, prior to Chiang's conversion to Christianity, Gale had provided supporters with evidence of an affinity between Nationalist forces and Christianity.

Educational efforts under the leadership of Mrs. Li, the wife of Gale's Tunki nurse, were presented as further evidence of this affinity, as it would apply toward Chinese women. Gale was one of many women missionaries who correlated Nationalist rule with the idea that Christianity could empower Chinese women.[69] As has been mentioned, Gale had linked the improved status of Chinese women with China's espousal of republican government. Moreover, missionaries believed that, since Nationalist leaders like Sun Yat-sen had been educated in mission schools, this movement's success would mean a boon for Christianity, which in turn would improve conditions for Chinese women.

Gale's existing correspondence to supporters does not indicate that much emphasis was placed upon Chinese women during the Tunki period, perhaps because she had been consumed with running and raising funds for her hospital. However, the attitude of the Gales toward womanhood, and Chinese women specifically, is revealed in Gale's praise for Mrs. Li in 1929 and in earlier correspondence to supporters.

In 1924, Francis Gale had reproached Tunki's male Chinese Christian church members because they did not consider letting their wives attend church services. According to his wife, the male Chinese Christians of Tunki believed their wives unworthy of the Christian message. Reverend Gale sought to change the men's minds: during one sermon, Francis Gale reminded the men of their wives' financial astuteness, the intelligence they demonstrated while running the family businesses and finances. Reverend Gale reasoned that if women were intelligent enough to accomplish these tasks, they could understand Christianity.

Gale's reiteration of her husband's message was significant because it emphasized that Chinese women's capabilities entitled them to attend church. Thus, the Gales did not insist that women attend church because it was morally right or because it was necessary in order to make them better caretakers. Rather, they emphasized that the intelligence of Chinese women rendered them worthy of the greater role Christianity offered.[70]

Mrs. Li was described by the Gales as an example of Nationalist faith in the intelligence of Chinese women, especially Christian women. The Nationalists had asked her to assist in instructing Tunki "women in matters consistent with good government." Gale described Mrs. Li as having been given "a place of honor" in the community until her death from tuberculosis in 1931. As Francis Gale noted, Nationalist support for Chinese Christian women helped improve the Tunki populace's attitude toward the Methodist Church.[71]

In short, Ailie Gale's message to supporters was that Tunki Nationalists respected Christians; and that if any Nationalist anti-Christian tendencies did surface, they were easily thwarted by astute and articulate Chinese Christians. Even when tragedy struck, it seemed to bode well for the popularity of Chinese Christian leaders.

Trouble came, not from Nationalists, but from two hundred bandits who burned the church and the entire business section of the city of Tunki to ashes in April 1929. Mr. Shen had negotiated with bandit leaders who had demanded money, jewelry, guns and ammunition, but despite his attempts, soon much of the city, with the exception of Gale's hospital, was in flames, and thousands of people were homeless. While the catastrophe caused about twenty million dollars in property damage, Gale told supporters that amidst this wreckage, a door had literally been "burnt open for" Mr. Shen's "preaching the Gospel." In the midst of negotiations between Shen and the bandits, the Chinese pastor has risen to prominence.[72]

During this time of crisis and apparent victory for Christianity, Gale had emphasized that Chinese Christians should remain independent leaders. "The foreign element" should not be introduced in any but the monetary way: "If the Chinese there can bring out of that awful calamity a Church in which they have had a major part in building they ought to have a fair chance to try it out."[73] In keeping with her emphasis on financial support, Gale simultaneously presented readers with a large request.

The hospital and homes outside the city had been untouched by the trouble; therefore, both could be built up to compensate for the city's damages. Mr. Shen, had risen to the occasion and became "a leader of the people." Consequently, he needed a building where he could implement his work, the cost of which would be about $2,500. By 1929, the hospital was temporarily without a doctor. Gale asked supporters to continue sending gifts so that when a Chinese doctor was found, that person could immediately begin working with pay. From 1927 to 1930, funds and boxes of items for Shen and Tunki mission work arrived regularly from New York, New Jersey, California and Idaho.[74]

While on furlough in 1930, the Gales continued fund-raising efforts, visiting Los Angeles and speaking to the many friends who had "been deeply interested in Tunki." They spoke in churches as far south as San Diego, California. There the Mission Hills Church had expressed interest in the medical work of Dr. Gale. Finally, in May 1931, Francis Gale made his way to meet old friends at the Simpson Church, while his wife stayed behind to save on transportation costs.

While the Gales had tried to strengthen ties to mission field supporters during their furlough, worldwide depression would make its mark upon the Tunki field's evangelical and educational work. By December 1931, one month after the return of the Gales to the Shanghai American School, the Board determined that, despite Ailie Gale's self-supporting medical successes, financial hardships dictated that it was no longer possible to support a mission station in Tunki. Gale was disappointed, insisting that many other places could have better been given up than the Tunki area, "where the people are so friendly and where Mr. Shen has made such deep impression on the people."[75]

Despite Gale's protests, by December 1931 the Methodist Board formally severed its ties to the Tunki field, one of many mission outposts that were closed due to severe financial constraints. Consequently, Gale dismantled her hospital, storing drugs, medical supplies and hospital beds at the Shanghai American School. By 1933, the Gales new destination would be the Nationalist capital of Nanking.[76]

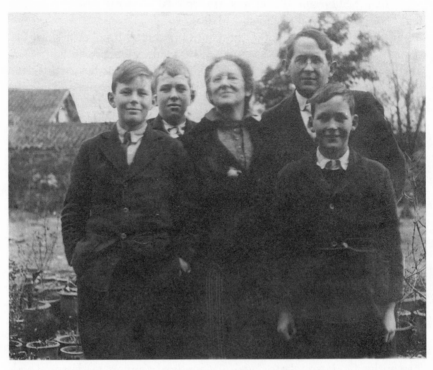

(Left to right) Lester, Spencer, Ailie, Francis Sr. and Francis Jr., in Nanchang (1910s).

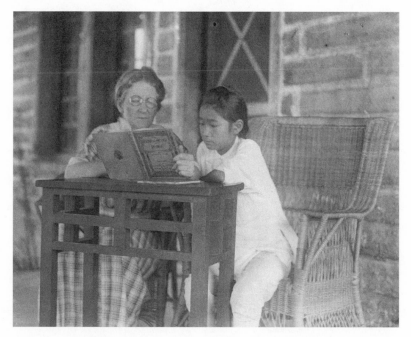

Gale giving English-language instruction to daughter Mary Gao (1910s).

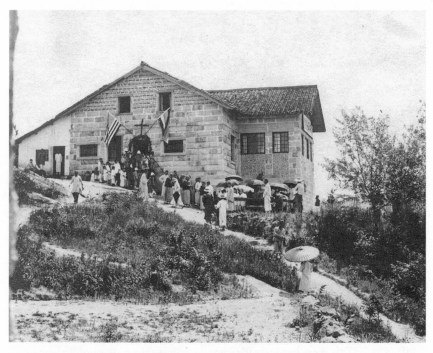

The exterior of Dr. Gale's eighteen-bed hospital, Tunki (1920s).

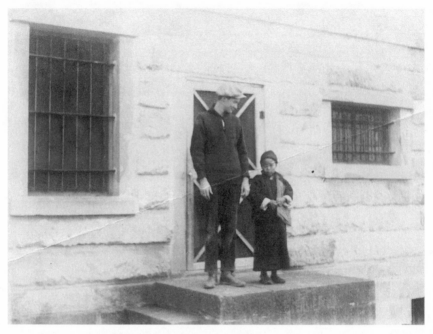

Frank Gale Jr. and Mary Gale (as a young child).

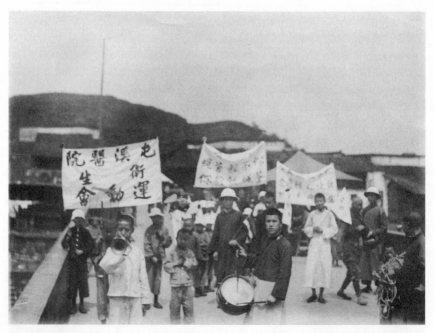

Tunki, 1926: With their bugles and drums, soldiers join Gale's public health parade.

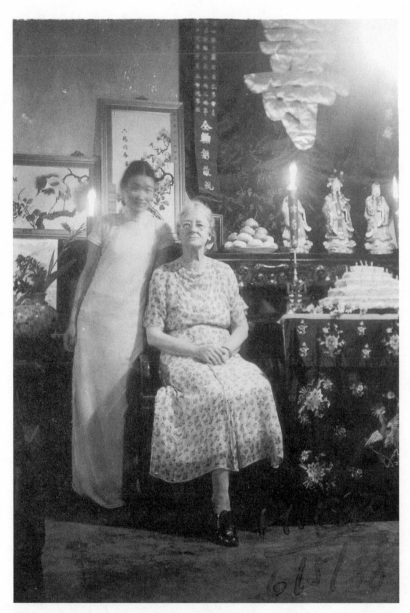

Mary Gao, standing at Ailie Gale's side.

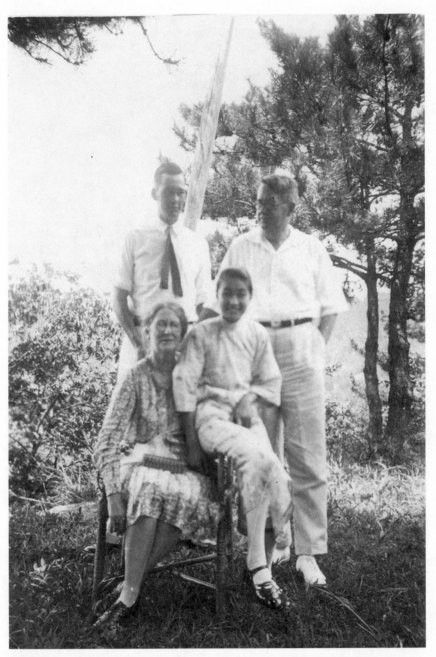

(Standing left to right): Frank Jr., Frank Sr., (Sitting left to right): Ailie Gale, Mary Gale.

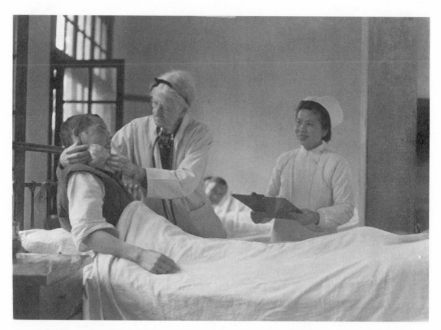
Dr. Ailie Gale treating a man injured by bandits (undated).

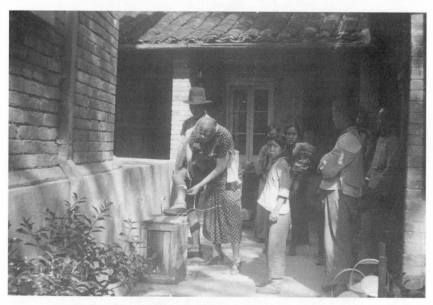
Dr. Ailie Gale's backdoor clinic, Nanking (1930s).

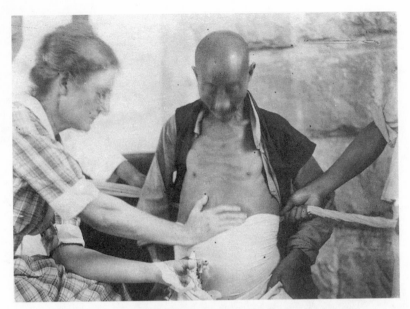

Dr. Ailie Gale removing fluid from a patient's stomach (undated).

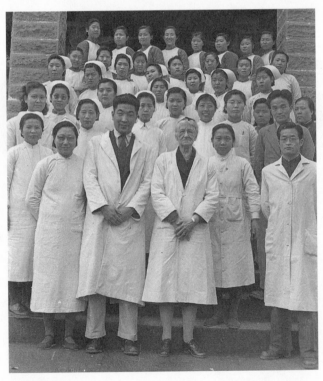

Dr. Ailie Gale and staff at Chadwick Memorial Hospital, Tzechung.

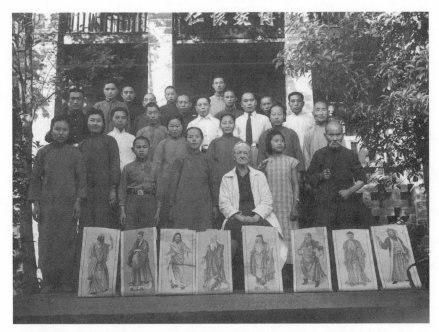

Dr. Ailie Gale (1940s).

6

Female Protestant Ideals, Liberal Protestantism, and Chinese Nationalist Ideology Converge in Nanking

WITH FORTY-ONE BOXED CRATES GATHERED FROM STORAGE IN THE Shanghai American School attic, Gale was en route to her new mission field in Nanking by 4 September 1933.[1] At the conclusion of her voyage up the Yangtze on a China Navigation Company steamer, Gale and her husband joined six other Methodist missionary couples at work in what had been the Nationalist government capital since 1927.[2] From 1933 to 1940, Gale established two clinics, and, under temporary contract with the WFMS, provided medical services for Chinese women at Ginling College,[3] a union institution run by women's Baptist, Methodist and Presbyterian societies.[4] Gale's clinics and work at Ginling, a continuation of her earlier focus on the medical, social and spiritual needs of the Chinese, typified women's missionary work. Prior to the 1930s, Gale's and the other women's work gained support from local Chinese officials and this doubtlessly had had an important impact on women missionaries' credibility with the home mission field. During the 1930s, women China missionaries gained greater status as women's ideals were incorporated into mainstream Liberal Protestantism and Nationalist government ideology. This chapter will focus upon how these two larger forces were intertwined with, and provided a positive context for, Gale's professional and personal achievements.

Gale's depictions of her professional successes as a medical missionary in her clinics and at Ginling College, and her relationship with, and influence on Chinese women, particularly her adopted daughter Mary, were a direct product of her belief in Christianity as a force for female empowerment. Gale portrayed women, including herself, as competent professionals who had an important public role. Broader forces such as Protestant China missionaries' increasing awareness and concern for the social and economic needs of China's poor, the Methodist Episcopal

Board of Mission's recognition of Gale's work with rural Chinese during the 1920s, and her association with the Nationalist government, gave even greater import to Gale's depiction of her professional success as a doctor. While these broader forces were influenced by other factors, such as the direct influence of Chinese Nationalists' protests, they also reflected the ways in which female Protestant ideals were propagated in China.[5]

The result of this fortuitous confluence was Gale's increased credibility with home mission field supporters in the United States during the 1930s, a time when the American public's sentimental attachment toward China became particularly strong. This chapter will illustrate how Gale's depictions of the Chinese Nationalists could spur supporter receptivity while simultaneously enhancing her own prestige.

Nationalist leader Chiang Kai-shek's marriage to Methodist Soong Meiling and conversion to Protestantism in 1931, had aroused much optimism among Protestant missionaries. This optimism was enhanced when Chiang issued his 1934 speech calling for a movement to achieve a new life for China.

Chiang's New Life Movement stemmed from his belief in the internal, highly militarized organization of Chinese society. By reaching deeply into the lives of individual Chinese, demanding patriotism and imposing draconian controls on their cleanliness and discipline, he argued that China could quickly elevate herself to Japan's and Germany's level of achievement. However, this was only one aspect of the Chiang's program for China.

In its efforts to answer both Communism's and Christianity's call for social reform, Chiang's movement competed with the aims of the "internal" menace, the "Red bandits." Simultaneously, Chiang would also appeal to Protestant missionaries, and women in particular.[6]

Scholars have emphasized the New Life Movement's amalgam of Fascism and Confucianism, and have perceived Christianity's contribution to it as an antipermissive Puritanism. However, the launching of the New Life Movement had been a challenge to Mao Tse-tung's Kiangsi land redistribution policies, and Chiang's desire to challenge Communism prompted him to begin to address the basic needs of the Chinese people. In the process, Chiang found a mode of convergence with the Protestant Christian missions' growing concern with the plight of rural Chinese. Consequently, and with some insistence from his wife, Chiang began to involve Protestant missionaries closely in his work.[7]

Like many Protestant missionaries, Gale would dismiss the importance of the New Life Movement's draconian qualities and instead place emphasis on its social programs for rural China. Like many women missionaries, Gale was preoccupied with the medical and social problems of the

Chinese and enthusiastic that the new Chinese government appeared to share these concerns. Gale's credibility with supporters was partially strengthened by her affirmations of the Nationalist government's apparent interest in the social needs of the Chinese people—a cause that, for decades, had served as an important bond in the relationship between women China missionaries and their female home field supporters.

Affinity of purpose between Gale and the Nationalists was compounded by her association with one of the movement's main Western advisors: the New Zealand-born, American-adopted, Congregationalist missionary George Shepherd, whom Chiang had singled out to help direct his movement. Moreover, Gale's credibility was enhanced as supporters learned of Shepherd's importance to the movement.

George Shepherd had been an evangelical missionary working in Northern Fukien when his work was curtailed by the Northern Expedition of 1927. As James Thomson has noted, Shepherd had had firsthand experience with the Communists during their brutal occupation of Kiangsi; however, Shepherd's reaction had been ambiguous. On the one hand, he was repulsed by the Communists' cruel excesses; on the other, Shepherd respected their attention to needs of the majority of rural Chinese, a matter which Chiang had previously ignored.[8]

Shepherd began to redirect his attention from traditional evangelical goals to a rural Christian program in 1931, when Mao Tse-tung established the Chinese Soviet Republic in Kiangsi and embarked upon a radical land redistribution program. Recognizing the value of his extensive experience and ideas for countering Communist appeal, Chiang appointed Shepherd to supervise a network of promotional associations which would implement the New Life Movement from the provincial to the hsien levels in the areas of Kiangsi seized from the Communists.[9]

The Kiangsi program was run by a team of experts, two executive secretaries, a Chinese and a missionary—all of whom trained native leaders to supervise village work in five areas: self-defense, connection to an agricultural experiment station, public health work with a nurse and a doctor, village industries, and religious training. Chiang's Special Movement Force recovered an area from the Communists, surveyed the needs of the people, lent assistance to families and maintained order until a local government could be set up. They carried on morality drives and mass education programs, addressing a myriad of social needs.[10]

Shepherd was in charge of teams of Chinese volunteers who were working for a small salary. Frequently shuttling from Nanking to South Fukien to gather money and workers, Shepherd was often in need of room and board. While in Nanking, he availed himself of the Gale home and in the process established a warm friendship with his hosts.

Gale's connection to Shepherd was cemented from 1934 and 1937, when Chiang's network of associations was particularly impressive, spanning nineteen provinces.[11] These associations extended farther than his effective military control. Consequently, Gale perceived a stronger nationalist leadership, and hence, Christian influence than was actually the case. The presumed strength of Chiang gave even greater import to George Shepherd's status as the one trusted American in the inner circle of Chiang Kai-shek and one of the closest of Madame Chiang's non-Chinese collaborators.[12] Gale profited from her friendship and the new celebrity status she gained by her company with George Shepherd. Beginning in 1934, her correspondence mentioned Shepherd's usage of the Gales' Nanking home and his vacations with them, and many other Protestant missionaries in the mountainous summer resort of Kuling, near Kiukiang.[13]

Due to his close relationship with Chiang and his wife, Gale considered Shepherd a better authority on China than any newspaper.[14] Gale thought she benefited from George Shepherd's knowledge of "matters of government."[15] She delighted in sitting at her kitchen table with Bishop Ralph Ward and Shepherd, discussing "world affairs."[16] Importantly, Gale respected Shepherd, declaring Chiang wise for having selected him to supervise a rural plan which she found appealing for China.[17] Gale's relationship with Shepherd was one important factor which enabled her to display confidence when informing supporters of political events in China.

Adding to Gale's prestige with supporters was the Methodist Episcopal Board's growing attention to the social needs of rural Chinese. The shift in the Methodist Episcopal Board of Missions' policy during the 1930s was no different from that of other Protestant Boards. An important impetus for this change in perspective were the catastrophic events that worsened the lot of rural Chinese, making their plight increasingly difficult to ignore: the flooding of the Yangtze and Huai Rivers during the summer of 1931 and the increasing impact of worldwide depression. In response to these developments, Protestant mission boards began to downplay evangelism and the creation of metropolitan institutions run by missionaries, and emphasized instead the social needs of China's poor, the turning over of missionary institutions to the Chinese, and the need for missionary work in rural areas. The Methodist Board's recognition of Gale's work suggests that women missionaries played a significant role in this shift.

Most Protestant foreign missionary boards' emphasis upon social gospel efforts and concern for rural China had begun in the late 1920s in response to the growing nationalist protests of the Chinese and the publication of such studies as the 1928 report of agricultural specialist Kenyon L. Butterfield. Butterfield recommended a "rural community parish," and by 1930, he had structured a specific social and economic program for China.[18]

The transformation that began during Gale's years in Tunki was not rapid. Historian James Thomson has noted that the delegates to the 1922 National Christian Conference decreed that Christians should give greater attention to the "social and physical welfare of the people to whom they preached." By 1927, however, there still were no clear advances made toward a coherent Protestant program for the Chinese countryside. That year, the report of the Conference on Christianizing Economic Relations, under the auspices of the National Christian Council of China, included ten pages of discussion on rural economic problems in contrast to the thirty pages devoted to industrial conditions.[19]

As Gale's work in Tunki had preceded Protestant missionary boards' organized efforts to attend to the social and physical needs of China's poor, it was hailed by the Methodist Episcopal board an the example to be followed. While Dr. J. G. Vaughan had previously taken exception to Gale's apparently open-minded attitude toward the Chinese (during their years together at Nanchang General Hospital) in early 1931, he expressed a change in perspective. Vaughan reported his, and other board members' growing sentiment that "missionary policy ought to lead us out from the big metropolitan centers to the smaller towns and villages where we will have a less institutional emphasis and closer contact with the people." Vaughan correctly noted that the first phase of missionary work had been characterized by the consolidation of Methodist institutions in metropolitan areas. These were considered "feeders for the outlying districts." He had come to believe that they should rightly be turned over to "Nationals, thus setting the missionaries free to go out into the towns and villages." Vaughan considered Dr. and Mr. Gale a "remarkable couple for this kind of work," with his "evangelistic zeal," and her "medical" and "intimate knowledge of the Chinese people." Thus while the board had been forced to shut down the Tunki mission field, they came to consider the Gales' work there as a model for "typical centers of this" sort.[20]

As has been noted, Gale's work had not only been typical as a guide for the future of mission work: it had been characteristic of women missionaries, most of whom had been attending to the social and physical needs of the Chinese since the mid-nineteenth century.[21] The Nationalist government's growing interest in this work, Gale's friendship with the influential George Sheperd, and the increasing numbers of social gospel practitioners and liberal missionaries in the China field, all provided validation for Gale's (and other women missionaries' work) and her supporters' long-standing interest in it.

Within the context of these broader forces, one can understand the significance of Gale's medical work in Nanking, and her continued emphasis upon the social and physical needs of the China's poor. While in Nanking, Gale forged an increasingly tighter link between supporter funds and the social needs of the poor while continuing to affirm her credibility and competence as both a physician and administrator. Upon arrival to Nanking, Gale reported that her usage of supporter funds enabled her to initiate medical work immediately. She had had the foresight to place the balance of supporters' contributions to the Tunki Hospital in a Shanghai bank which had weathered the financial difficulties through which most banking institutions in China had succumbed.[22]

Gale used the funds to paint and purchase medical supplies and furniture for a clinic for the poor in a Methodist Church located in a densely populated area of downtown Nanking, then a city of 400,000. Gale explained that she had chosen this site because, while government clinics were growing rapidly, there was none in that vicinity.[23] Throughout her stay, supporter funds paid for Gale's treatment of Nanking's poorest citizens, such as rickshaw coolies and others who found government hospital fees too high, and Chinese pastors and Bible women.[24]

As in Nanchang and Tunki, Gale's credibility with the home field was enhanced during these years by her reports of successes with complex medical procedures requiring high skill. Pastor Shen frequently brought Gale ailing and poor church members with a myriad of needs. Gale told supporters that her duties encompassed mastoid and eye operations, as well as psychiatric care.[25]

As in the past, much of Gale's work gave supporters validation for a feminized medicine, emphasizing preventative care and the patient's total well being. Gale expressed the typical womanly concern with the whole patient, not just the disease. She emphasized the physical, spiritual, and intellectual needs of patients, linking these to their good health and well being. Gale perceived her medical duties as intertwined with the English, mathematics, and music classes and Boy's Clubs held in the Methodist church building, noting: "It seems fitting that medical work should go along with these varied activities."[26]

By late 1936, Gale's medical work was confined only to Ginling, two Methodist Bible Schools and a "back-door" clinic she ran from her home. Gale reported that she happily stopped the medical work at the Nanking Methodist Church clinic when the nurse there became sufficiently able to treat most cases. Leaving her nurse in charge, Gale treated only those in severe need: the poor, usually from families of nearly destitute rickshaw men, in the immediate vicinity of her home. These individuals could not "spare the few coppers needed to go to one of the public health centers," according to Gale. Supporters' monies helped pay for medicine and serums for vaccinations dispensed at these clinics; and, as in the past, Gale's reports of appreciation for work enhanced her credibility and insured the continuation of contributions.[27]

Gale's greatest love, taking up the largest portion of her day, was public health work. Three days a week, from 8:30 A.M. to 6:00 P.M., Gale held a clinic at Ginling College. She gave the patients inoculations for cholera and typhoid,[28] and during one week in 1934 she performed three hundred physical exams, working from early morning until five in the afternoon. "My head was so weary that I could scarcely think," she wrote to her sons, noting that there were twenty more examinations remaining to be done.[29]

Gale not only practiced feminized medicine, but also taught it to her students at Ginling. For example, in 1934 Gale assisted Ginling College's Sociology majors with a public health project which was both educational and of immediate social value. The Ginling girls were in charge of selecting eight amahs and overseeing their feeding and care of eight babies from a nearby orphanage. Gale studied the ingredients in Carnation milk, constructed a table for infant feeding, and apportioned the list of ingredients in the milk to the ages and weights of each of the babies.[30] At Ginling, Gale was not only a physician, but also an educator and social worker. Of most importance to women home field supporters, Gale presented herself as an influential role model in the lives of young Chinese women.

Gale informed supporters that she was accepted and respected at Ginling. According to Rev. Gale, by June 1934, his wife had already "won a large place in the hearts of" Ginling colleagues and students. Proof of this came when a Ginling nurse died a tragic and untimely death that year and Gale was given the honor of giving a eulogy at the service. Reverend Gale noted that the audience was impressed with his wife's talk.[31]

Gale was comfortable speaking to Ginling faculty and students because she described the school's atmosphere as one which fostered the type of role Gale believed women should have. Gale's description of Ginling students provided women supporters with the knowledge that the college's faculty and its Nationalist government supporters hoped for a large public role for the emerging modern Chinese woman.

Ginling College graduated China's first women college students in 1919. The school's motto was "Abundant Life," and its purpose was to "offer special courses in premedical sciences, in education," and "in religion, fitting women students for service in the three fields of ministry to the needs of body, mind and spirit."[32]

In 1934, Gale described Nationalist officials' support of the school to friends at the Simpson Church, when she forwarded a pamphlet depicting a dedication service for a New Library and Chapel Buildings at the College. At the ceremony, the Nationalist Minister of Education, Wang Shih-chi, told the audience that he believed college women had a role that went beyond the domestic and personal realm: they should be "economically productive and not educated merely to raise their own standard of living" but ultimately, they should "take the lead in all worthy movements for the reconstruction of China." Dr. Wu, the President of Ginling College, emphasized that modern day circumstances gave Chinese women the obligation to "cultivate their minds." Wu believed that these circumstances created opportunities that offered women equality with men.[33]

Gale had expressed discomfort with the young American women at the Shanghai American School a few years earlier, but she often expressed her affinity with Ginling's young college women. Perhaps because she felt that they might be more willing to follow her direction than American women, Gale not only enjoyed working with them, but frequently invited them to her home for breakfast and dinner.[34] Despite her desire to replace their culture with her own, Gale's comments suggested that she admired her students. As she told supporters, the girls were the most talented in China, hand-picked from high schools all over the nation, and she hoped her influence upon them would reach "beyond the medical."[35]

Gale had appeared reserved to many young girls at the Shanghai American School, but her attitude toward life reflected Chinese casualness, rather than Western prudishness: she believed in educating young women regarding spousal selection, love and the intimate details of married life.[36] On one occasion, when Ginling students visited Gale for an evening of Victrola records, the girls had asked to hear the details of Dr. and Rev. Gale's engagement period and the couple's engagement song. They had also asked one guest, a single female missionary, for an account of her "love affairs."[37] Gale was happy to note that the women "seemed to enjoy" the discussion. Her evaluation of the evening's discourse was: this is "new China and not the one we found when we came."[38]

Gale believed that women's missionary work had already made an impact upon Chinese women. During a banquet given by the senior class at Ginling College in 1935, Gale observed that Chinese girls had put on a fun show of Spanish, Swedish, and Irish dances. She compared their ease and agility to earlier conditions: in Nanchang, the girls had had bound feet and during one public performance, "they put foreign shoes on over their little silk ones," covering their "queer looking feet." Inadvertently revealing her disdain for traditional Chinese culture, Gale contrasted the "very stilted forms of calisthenics" of years past with the program put on by the Ginling girls, remarking: "Such a program would have scandalized the city. . . . What changes twenty five years can make."[39]

By 1936, Gale appealed to supporters by showing not only that Chinese women had come a long way, but also that their gratitude could result in economic support. In a Christmas letter to friends, Gale described the dedication of the Ginling College's new infirmary, designed in accordance with Gale's specifications. She recalled: "While I was at the American School in Shanghai, realizing the need of a properly equipped infirmary, I had spent much thought on the kind of building that would meet the needs," but Gale could not implement her goal at the time.[40]

In response to a request from Gale, the President of Ginling, Dr. Wu, had sent out a letter to some of the college's alumnae asking for contributions to finance the construction of an infirmary building designed in accordance with her wishes. Shortly thereafter, the alumnae raised eleven thousand dollars for the building and equipment. Gale remarked that the finished product was "quite complete for the purpose for which it was built."[41] Chinese women had shown their willingness to support a Western woman. In addition, they also demonstrated that they had the power to provide full economic support for the building at the institution that embodied core female Protestant missionary ideals: Ginling College.

The most tangible proof of Gale's wish to influence Chinese women was her depiction of her adopted Chinese daughter Mary. Gale had adopted Mary and raised her to speak and write Mandarin, dress Chinese, and look forward to serving her country. Until mid-1934, Mary appeared to absorb her mother's ideals of mental cultivation and female empowerment, but then she rebelled against her mother. In the eventual resolution of this conflict, one can see the extent of Gale's attitude toward and goals for Chinese women.

In April 1934, Gale proudly reported to supporters that Mary, whose nursing education was two-thirds completed, was asking important questions in order to decide how to personally meet the needs of Chiang Kai-shek's New Life Program.[42] However, as soon as this enthusiasm appeared to reach its peak, Mary began to rebel against her mother's conceptions of womanhood: at the age of twenty-two, she decided to become its antithesis.

In September 1934, Gale reported that Mary no longer wished to continue her nursing studies at the Wuhu Hospital. She had developed a friendship with another female nurse, and both women rebelled against the hospital authorities, failing to meet their required nursing duties. Mary went on a hunger strike, lost an alarming amount of weight in protest and begged to return home to her parents in Nanking for a hiatus from nursing.[43]

Gale not only despaired at Mary's rebellion, but also at what she viewed as a despondency toward life. She lamented that Mary returned home to her parents, surrounded by great literature, yet she never picked up a book. Gale complained of Mary's preoccupation with knitting (a domestic endeavor) and her aversion to newspapers (a typically male concern by traditional standards). Perplexed at Mary's ignorance of current events, Gale noted: "She had not the faintest idea who Mussolini was."[44] Gale described her daughter as "listless . . . that one wonders if she will ever take enough interest in anything to make a success of it."[45] Francis Gale complained that Mary was child-like in her impudence, taking issue with even the smallest parental request and pouting for hours when she did not get her way.[46]

By December 1934, however, Mary's rebellion was over and she seemed determined to pursue the kind of public service career that Gale had encouraged. Gale's letters to supporters would explain neither Mary's rebellion nor its cessation. Evidently a compromise had been struck, as Mary completed her nurse's training at the Nanking University Hospital. A poor recommendation from her former employer dictated that she begin in the Nanking hospital's diet kitchen, but Mary worked hard at paying her dues and hoped soon to get back into regular nursing duties.[47]

Anxious to present Mary in a favorable light, Gale was selective about what she told supporters at the Simpson Church concerning her daughter's ordeal. Gale emphasized Mary's physical illness and weak constitution, explaining that she was temporarily given a secretarial job until she was able to put on some weight and regain the strength needed to go back to regular nursing work at the hospital.[48]

Conversely, Gale's descriptions of Mary's recovery and invigorated enthusiasm for public service work spared no details. By 1936, Gale reported proudly that Mary was "very keen on the Public Health work and thinks now she wants to specialize" in that field. According to Gale, Mary was "very enthusiastic" and looked "like a different girl from the one who came home from Wuhu." Gale's letters detailed Mary's hard work and future goals: "She vaccinated 139" during just one day on the job and had plans to take a more intensive course in public health.[49]

By August 1936, Gale proudly explained to Simpson Church supporters that Mary had complied with a Nationalist government regulation that all student nurses take three months of Public Health training, immediately finding that this field was her calling. As a public health nurse, Mary was assigned to study the occupation, salary, debts and interest owed by Nanking's poor.[50] By December 1936, Gale's quarterly letter to supporters declared that Mary was "now a graduate nurse . . . planning to specialize in Public Health." As though eager to provide more tangible proof of Mary's new status, she promised the Simpson Church a picture of her daughter in her nurse's uniform, a deep blue, with white collar and cuffs.[51] A few months later, Gale reported that Mary believed herself as knowledgeable as a doctor, and expressed the wish for further study in the United States.[52]

Mary's work ethic was a testimony to her mother's values: public service took priority, and its success hinged on her ability to cultivate her talents and develop her skills. While Mary's decision to pursue public service, a typically womanly endeavor, may have seemed like a boon to traditional women's values, Mary had not been raised to become a conventional woman. While an excellent nurse, Mary was also a talented leader and administrator. Gale noted that she was assertive, complementing her nursing skills with the ability to get people to do what she wanted.[53]

Further, Mary's know-how and self-confidence reflected a growing personal independence. In March 1937, Gale noted that Mary had watched a movie called "The White Parade," in which a "nurse gave up her lover for [her] profession." Gale queried Mary for her reaction to the movie and when Mary responded that she "thought she ought to be that kind," her mother approved. Remembering the difficult time Mary had had at Wuhu in 1934, Gale concluded that her daughter had evidently "done some deep thinking."[54]

Gale had taught Mary that public service work not only took priority over marriage, but entitled her to express interest in and participate in the male-identified public realm: Gale was relieved when Mary put down her knitting needles and began to immerse herself in Chinese politics. In fact, Mary had become an avid reader of newspapers and was "quite up on the war situation," an expression of her more public orientation. As Gale observed: Mary was a "very patriotic young lady."[55]

In 1938, as Gale worked hard to understand political events in China, she wrote of her increasing admiration for Mary, who seemed to have the answers: "She is full of fine ideas and has eyes that see everything." Gale admitted that Mary "puts me wise on many things."[56]

Gale's descriptions of rapidly modernizing Chinese women, her work with and observations of Ginling students, and the empowered woman Mary had become, were all important to her representation to American women mission field supporters. In America, during the first half of the twentieth century, successful professional women were often depicted as unfeminine, unattractive and undesirable.[57] Gale and the Chinese women she influenced were independent professionals who might marry but did not necessarily need a man in order to be happy. They were doubtlessly not perceived by supporters as unattractive and mannish because they adhered to typically female values of social service. As in the nineteenth century, women's proclivity toward social concern represented a possibility to negotiate a measure of power in what was traditionally the male realm.[58]

During the 1930s, Gale's achievements may be viewed as a window to a broader confluence. There was the growth of a centrist Liberal Protestant majority, combined with the shift away from evangelism and the building of missionary-directed institutions and toward an increasing emphasis upon the social and economic needs of the Chinese. In this context, Chinese Nationalists' validation of women missionaries' ideology strengthened the import of Gale's representation as a credible, successful doctor.

During the 1930s, the meanings understood by women supporters to be essential to Gale's work and "empowerment-through-piety," facilitated Gale's description of the new direction for Protestant missionary work, the elevation of Chinese women and the role of Chinese Nationalists in fostering plans which reflected values that were accepted by many Protestant women. These factors enhanced Gale's credibility, rendering her a representative figure for the expansion of Western and Chinese women's roles during the 1930s. As has been noted, Gale's self-representation as an achiever was in direct proportion to her success at imparting information to supporters, a factor of paramount importance during the 1930s, when political struggles prompted Americans to question the wisdom of involvement in a China plagued by war. While Gale's correspondence to the United States reflected her public health work and work with women, following along patterns established in Nanchang and Tunki, these political struggles led Gale to alter the contents of her letters. Expressing faith in her judgment, American supporters frequently queried her for information concerning political developments there. By 1937, she noted that "almost every letter from U.S.A. asks some question about the political situation in China."[59]

Gale's response was to supply supporters with facts that would help them shape their opinions regarding developments in the Chinese civil war, Sino-Japanese war, and Sino-American alliance. Thus, beginning in Gale's Nanking years, a significant portion of her letters, both to supporters and family, were devoted to her observations of the war-time situation and the cast of characters struggling for power in China during the precarious 1930s.

7

Empowered by Piety, Victorious in War

WHEN THE COLORADO COLLEGE STUDENT NEWSPAPER, *THE TIGER*, reported the former Ailie Spencer's arrival on campus in March of 1941, they proudly noted her celebrity status, as evidenced by the numerous sight-seeing tours and teas arranged in her honor. The article remarked upon aspects of Gale that had inspired home mission field support for many years: she was an American-trained physician who had been supervisor of several hospitals in China for thirty-two years. The article asserted her expertise in the male-dominated international realm, noting that Gale was "very well informed as to the political condition of China." Further, she was deemed as courageous as she was worldly. Although her former post in Nanking was occupied by the Japanese, she was nonetheless undeterred from returning to the mission field: she would take the Burma Road and looked forward to "rough[ing] it" in her new post in Western China.[1]

At her former alma mater in Colorado Springs, Gale gave talks, reiterating information doubtlessly repeated since the beginning of her furlough in the United States in April 1940. *The Tiger* described Gale's assessment of the Sino-Japanese war as very "optimistic." She reported that Japanese occupation of China had required the westward relocation of all of China's educational institutions; however, Gale reminded Americans that most of the cultural centers had not been destroyed, but rather, moved, a crucial symbol of China's capacity for endurance.[2] Indeed, the content of Gale's lecture at her former college echoed that of her correspondence to supporters and family during the 1930s, a time when, as historian John Dower notes, most Americans failed to "take the Japanese seriously" in their ability to conquer China.[3]

American optimism over China's ability to withstand Japanese aggression stemmed in great part from the communications of missionaries to their home field supporters. As historian Paul Varg has noted: "From the time of the Manchurian Incident of 1931 to Pearl Harbor, the American

Protestant missionaries in China dedicated themselves to enlightening the home constituency."[4]

Public perceptions of the Sino-Japanese struggles of the 1930s and 1940s eventually made a significant impact upon the formation of United States's foreign policy in World War II. By the time Franklin D. Roosevelt began to publicly identify Japan as a national security threat, he found American public opinion a fertile ground for his desired pro-China policy.[5] Missionaries like Gale had contributed to the creation of this amenable atmosphere.

Gale's writings during the 1930s, and talks while on furlough in 1940 and 1941, provide a view of how one American missionary projected the Chinese as capable of eventually achieving victory over their presumably stronger military opponents. Gale's interpretation also helps one understand how some women missionaries' perceptions and interpretations of the Sino-Japanese war stemmed from their religious ideals.

In her correspondence to supporters, Gale suggested that piety could empower, not only other women, but also races and nations, rendering people of all races equals. Gale often expressed a horizontal, rather than a vertical or hierarchical, worldview that while Christians of all genders and races were superior to non-Christians, Chinese and Westerners, like men and women, should work side by side. These assertions were understood by women supporters, as the language mirrored that of nineteenth-century Protestant women missionary workers who had subverted male power by asserting their obligation to serve God alongside their male counterparts.

Despite this, Gale's public expressions must be balanced with, and understood alongside her actual China experience. Gale was a cultural imperialist in her unwavering insistence that the Chinese needed to replace their religious beliefs with Christianity, a Western import. While professing the need for cooperation, she consistently placed herself in a position of power, where she delegated, rather than accepted, orders to both white and Chinese men and women. Gale did not question her own nation's, or Western political dominance over China in general. Moreover, the belief that Christianity could empower did not render Gale's reaction to Japanese imperialism either predictable or unchanging. Given these contradictions, however, this chapter will examine how the Gale's belief in Christianity as a force for empowerment, led her to describe the Sino-Japanese conflict from the late 1920s and 1930s to the bombing of Pearl Harbor in 1941, and how she portrayed the fighting in her correspondence to family and supporters in the United States.

As has been noted, when confronted with protests against Japanese imperialism in Tunki, Anhwei, Gale favored directing the Chinese toward what she believed to be more productive endeavors such as public health, reasoning that this was energy better spent.[6] However, when her years at the Shanghai American School coincided with the 1927 ascendancy of the Nationalist regime and its efforts to regain Chinese influence from the Japanese in Manchuria, Gale began to sympathize with Chinese protests. After a one-year furlough ending in August 1931, Gale would return to Shanghai in time for the onset of Japanese military efforts to establish a base in Northeast China.

The Japanese army and navy believed their nation's economic self-sufficiency and national security hinged upon a sphere of influence in Manchuria. Since their 1895 victory over China, Japanese railway investments and interests in Manchuria's rich resources had steadily increased. Taking advantage of China's factious state and the cooperation of Northern Chinese warlords, the Japanese had dominated Manchuria's rich coal deposits and the South Manchurian Railway; however, in the mid-1920s, Japanese influence was threatened by both the Soviet Union and Chiang Kai-shek's attempts to reclaim north China.[7]

In response to Chiang, the Japanese began protecting their interests, by sending an armed expedition to Tsinan in 1927. Later, when Manchurian warlord Chang Tso-lin turned his back on an important rail expansion project with the Japanese to form an alliance with the Nationalists, he was assassinated by a Japanese army officer. Lack of cooperation from the warlord's son prompted Japanese army officers to eventually set off a small explosion near the South Manchurian Railway in September 1931, blame it on the Chinese, and send forces into Chichihar. By March 1932, the Japanese military had not only established the new state of Manchukuo, but also set the stage for the future conflict with China.[8]

With her relocation from Tunki to Shanghai in 1927, Gale had been introduced to a cosmopolitan city bristling with anti-Japanese hostility. Four years later, Gale returned from furlough in the United States to an even more tension-filled Shanghai. Anti-Japanese sentiment was manifested not only in the standard student demonstrations, speeches, and boycotts Gale had seen in 1927, but also with the organization of an anti-Japanese militia.[9]

These forms of Chinese protest elicited strong Japanese reaction. Japanese businessmen were hurt by the boycotts and demanded that their military authorities take action. Eager to respond to Chinese aggression, Japanese ultranationalists, Kwantung Army leaders, and the Japanese navy independently plotted to create another incident.[10]

In January 1932, when a Sino-Japanese clash in a towel factory resulted in Japanese injuries and one death, these angry Japanese groups got their wish. Shanghai's Japanese naval commander used this as a pretext for stringent demands: compensation for Japanese victims and an agreement from the mayor of Shanghai, Wu T'ieh-ch'eng, to evacuate Chinese military units thirty li from the Shanghai area (one li is about equal to 1/3 mile).[11]

Motivated by the belief that China's conventional army was inferior to that of the Japanese, that only appeasement would slow down China's invaders, and that Chinese forces should fight Communists before the Japanese, Chiang ordered Wu T'ieh-ch'eng to avoid conflict with Japan at all costs. Chiang formally proclaimed this view in March 1932 with the doctrine of "achieving internal pacification before resisting foreign aggression," to which he firmly adhered until 1937.[12]

Despite Chiang's new appeasement strategy and Wu T'-ieh-ch'eng's determination to comply, the local Chinese military force, the Cantonese Nineteenth Route Army, refused to yield to Japanese encroachment.[13] On 28 January 1932, these tough, independent soldiers began their brave fight with Japanese marines in Chapei, a poor residential section of Shanghai.

No fighting took place near the Shanghai American School, located in the French concession, but the experiences and understandings Gale acquired in Shanghai during this period of conflict began to shape her views and interpretation of the Sino-Japanese War. At the school, Gale helped students prepare suitcases and led the school's frequent evacuation drills. Gale saw protective sandbags, barbed wire, and defense perimeters patrolled by soldiers. She heard first-hand reports of Japanese atrocities against Chinese civilians and destruction of Chinese property.[14] Importantly, her presence during the "Shanghai incident" helped Gale formulate the impression that would remain with her throughout the Sino-Japanese War: the Chinese were brave, astute fighters, capable of outwitting their attackers no matter how formidable their Japanese opponents. In 1932, Gale's impression had a strong basis in reality.

When the 6,000 Japanese marines came face to face with the Chinese army of 20,000, they expected immediate victory. However, not even incendiary bombs, advanced artillery, and tanks could dislodge the Cantonese Army. Japanese army divisions were brought in and reinforcements rose on both sides.[15]

Brutal escalation resulted because unexpected Chinese tenacity had threatened a defeat that the Japanese military could not afford to allow. In the end, the Japanese established air superiority over the battle zone and the Japanese navy remained on the Yangtze. However, Shanghai's Chinese defenders had become heroes, and their spirit came to be synonymous with Chinese stoicism throughout the Sino-Japanese War.[16]

Historians such as Paul Varg have noted that missionary depictions of the Sino-Japanese struggle emphasized the portrayal of Japan "as a militaristic nation, callous to all humanitarian considerations, bent on reducing China to a servile status."[17] Varg's account reflects scholarly attention to accounts which portray China as weak, victimized, and in need of mothering.[18] However, beginning in 1931 with the Manchurian Incident, Gale's perceptions are significant for their emphasis upon the strength, incremental successes, and resilience of the Chinese, rather than upon their victimization by a stronger power.

Gale's optimism is not surprising: she had endeavored to provide readers with a positive portrayal of the Chinese since her arrival in 1908. Chinese respect and support for Gale and her professional endeavors, after all, had enhanced her own credibility with supporters. Moreover, during wartime, when strength was the criteria for success, the momentous events of late 1931 and early 1932 led Gale to identify the Cantonese Army's brave resistance to the revival of Chinese determination and spirit, which had been broken by the loss of Manchuria.[19] While these fighters had been at odds with Chiang Kai-shek's goal of appeasing the Japanese, Gale projected their perseverance and military prowess to qualities inherent to the Chinese, linking these to the ability of Chiang's forces to withstand the Japanese throughout the remainder of the war.

Gale began to project a tough and war-ready Chinese nation at the onset of Chiang's series of "local" settlements with Japanese officials in the north. The treaty of Tangku marked the first step in Chiang's three-year policy of "first pacification" and his efforts to strike a delicate balance between cooperating with Japan and squelching the influence of the anti-Japanese men in his midst.[20] The Japanese crossed the Great Wall in May 1933, and the Tangku Treaty left them in control of the area to its north, providing for a demilitarized zone marked by a railway line running between there and Peking.[21]

Beginning in 1934, supporters learned from Gale that the militarily astute Chinese were unafraid of conflict with Japan. While privately expressing sadness at Chinese military "blunders" and "careless bombing," the accidental attack on the ill-fated American ship, the *Hoover*, and the consequent death and injury of 1,500 civilians, Gale simultaneously evinced optimism. She argued that these errors did not reflect overall Chinese capabilities. Rather, it seemed to Gale that, in the long run, the Chinese were simply too clever and resolute to allow the Japanese to succeed in their drive to reach Nanking.[22]

Privately, Gale doubted the breadth of Christianity among Nationalists.[23] However, these doubts were often supplanted by Gale's assertion that China had the power necessary for victory because of its Christian leaders.[24]

Gale's perception of the general pervasiveness of Christian influence in China prevented her from completely acknowledging Chiang's reluctance to expend military strength upon the Japanese in order to win control of his country. Throughout 1934, Chiang continued to placate the Japanese while moving forward with a Fifth Extermination Campaign against the Communists. Privately, and through discussion, Chiang controlled conflicts with the Japanese.[25] While Gale was aware of Chiang's unwillingness to fight the Japanese, her letters to supporters focused predominantly upon evidence of China's unity and determination to fight the external enemy under Chiang.

In the fall of 1934, Gale reported excitement in Nanking "with the arrival of military General Chiang Kai-shek" as "all sorts of maneuvers" went on in his benefit. Planes dropped fake bombs and other military demonstrations were held, keeping Gale and others on the alert. Gale reasoned that China's aggressive war preparations, evidence of support for their Christian leader, constituted proof that it was not weak and ripe for domination, as the Japanese argued.[26]

In part, Gale's descriptions of Chinese unity and war-mindedness were an effort to counter Japanese reports that China was weak and in chaos. Rather, she sought to inspire the American public's protests to their government, and American involvement and support for the Chinese.[27] She reasoned that if America had not been "selfish" and had called an economic boycott at the time of the Manchukuo incident, Japanese aggression in China would have been curtailed much earlier.[28] Correctly perceiving that United States Secretary of State Cordell Hull was not in favor of assisting the Chinese Nationalists, Gale lamented his unwillingness to suggest sanctions and push the Japanese out of North China. Gale believed that the American public could and should influence policy. Moreover, she wished American students would demand sanctions against Japan or any country that dared invade another.[29]

Gale's projections of Chiang's effective leadership went beyond her desire to influence policy. She projected Chiang as effective because she perceived him a Christ figure. Gale often described his fearless demeanor in the face of danger, the frequent Bible and prayer meetings he held, and his perennial spiritual serenity. Convinced of Chiang's eventual success, and with it, the triumph of Christianity, Gale explained many of Chiang's military failures as temporary, and caused by two factors: the presence of disloyal men, and Chiang's firm adherence to humanitarian, and Christian inspired, goals over immediate victory.

Gale's naive interpretation stood in stark contrast with Chiang's actual leadership strategies and limited power. Until 1937, Chiang's military hold had been tenuous and strained, his core beliefs at odds with much of the Chinese public. Of the twenty-three Chinese provinces, Chiang exercised effective control over only eleven by 1935.[30] From an ideological and practical perspective, Chiang's views had earned him many enemies. The Shanghai incident had unleashed an enraged Chinese public that demanded a tough resistance to Japan. The formidable Nineteenth Route Army and their supporters had believed in mobilizing and recruiting the masses to fight the Japanese, uniting both Manchuria and Shanghai, and making a clear distinction between what Chiang called the "Japanese bandits" and the "red bandits."[31]

Conversely, Chiang Kai-shek had distrusted mass movements, favoring the removal of both kinds of "bandits" by the draconian organization of society. Believing that his military forces did not equal Japan's, he had been willing to accept the loss of North China, acquiesce to the Japanese and focus his energies on organizing the country from the inside.

Gale downplayed evidence of Chiang's unwillingness to fight the Japanese because of her perception of China's Christian empowerment and eventual victory. However, this predisposition did not preclude her from developing a growing awareness of those who were frustrated with Chiang's stubborn refusal to fight the "external bandits."

One important reason for Gale's increasing understanding was the respect she had for her daughter Mary. Gale noted that Mary was, like many students, sympathetic to the plight of the Chinese Communists. As has been noted, Gale admitted that she had much to learn from her daughter.[32]

In addition, as early as 1926, Gale had witnessed first-hand Communism's appeal to the Chinese. In September of that year Gale went to her first Medical Association Conference in Peking. Feng Yu-hsiang, a warlord famous for switching his political affiliations, had been to Peking during his alliance with Communist Russia, shortly before the arrival of Gale.[33]

Although by the time Gale arrived in 1926, Feng had left, Peking residents still remembered his troops' brief occupation with apparent fondness. While in Peking, Gale spoke with pastors, shopkeepers and other city residents, noting with surprise that most people favored the "reds" on the basis of their experience with Feng. Peking residents explained that when Feng Yu-hsiang's soldiers were in Peking they treated people "unusually well and the shopkeepers did a thriving business." When Feng's soldiers were replaced by another group, conditions deteriorated; consequently, Peking residents anxiously awaited Feng's return, as Gale explained to supporters.[34]

The views of Gale's daughter and Peking residents had influenced her understanding of the Chinese Communists. In addition, two other factors led Gale to develop some awareness of Communism's appeal for poor Chinese. War and the economic distresses of the Chinese had prompted Gale to write more frequently about Nanking's poor as she provided them with medical treatment in her clinics.[35] Moreover, with Chiang's efforts to modernize Nanking, the Gales' street was renovated and they were rendered temporarily homeless. In October 1934, Chiang Kai-shek issued a decree that the streets of the city of Nanking be widened. Chiang promised to provide the city with one-third of the funds necessary; however, he ordered the buildings on the street on which the Gales' lived be torn down to fulfill a plan for widening three other streets. In protest, the Gales appealed to Nanking authorities.[36] It was in vain: as Gale told supporters on 10 November 1934, all of the churches, schools, homes and trees in the path of the military, would come down in response to the order of city officials.

The Methodists and Presbyterians lost two small churches but no foreign residence, but since the Gale home was the only foreign home to come down, they felt especially victimized. The Gales informed supporters that the Nationalist government would not assume the cost of rebuilding a new residence and would not pay for any of the land taken from others. Moreover, the government gave only a portion, twenty dollars, for the cost of the house the Gales lost: a small consolation. In a tone that was far from sympathetic to the new Nanking regime, Francis Gale asked supporters: "Do you wonder that many poor people who have lost land and buildings have committed suicide rather than face a life of begging?"[37]

An overview of Gale's experiences illustrates that she had ample reason to both sympathize with the Chinese Nationalists, who promised a victory for Christianity, and understand the appeal of Communism to a people she had come to love and respect. These experiences dictated Gale's response to the kidnapping of Chiang Kai-shek in late 1936.

When Gale initially learned of Chiang's kidnapping she was confused by the turn of events.[38] Anxious to be accurate and informative to supporters "since almost every letter from the U.S.A. (asked) some question about the political situation in China," Gale decided to postpone her quarterly letter until the return of her highly informed friend, George Shepherd.[39] Shepherd had spoken to Madame Chiang for many hours regarding the grievances of her husband's kidnappers, and he related his knowledge to the Gales. The information that Gale passed on to family and supporters reflected both Gale's and Shepherd's ambiguous perception of the Chinese Communists.

From Shepherd, Gale learned that Chang Hsueh-liang, a former opium addict, was reportedly a trusted friend of Chiang's. However, his men were from the north and wanted to return to Manchuria. They were frustrated because Chiang forced them to fight their fellow countrymen, rather than drive out the Japanese who were occupying their territory in north China.[40]

Chang Hsueh-liang had had much cause for grievance: the Japanese had killed his father in 1928 and his army had been driven out of Manchuria in 1931. Chang's frustration was further compounded when he lent his military expertise to the task of wiping out the Communist soviet in the Hopei-Henan-Anhui border area and the Japanese became even more aggressive. They made plans to establish an independent regime in Inner Mongolia and extend the demilitarized zones established during the Tangku truce to all of Hopei province.[41]

Gale's February 1937 letter to supporters reflected both George Shepherd's insider's account of the events surrounding the Sian Incident, Gale's own varied experiences, and frustration at simplistic American reports of the China scene. In particular, Gale took issue with *Time* magazine's coverage of the incident.

Gale concurred with *Time*'s support of Chiang's previous efforts to concentrate his military strength against the Chinese Communists. However, she complained that the magazine's summary of the episode did not acknowledge the valid claims of the large numbers of Chinese who protested Chiang's refusal to fight the Japanese. Gale was aware that many students, including her own daughter Mary, did not support Chiang because he fought his own countrymen. Consequently, Gale's perception of *Time*'s summary of the Sian Incident was that it was "not true by any stretch of the imagination" because it had failed to explain that "on the side of the rebels, there were many causes for discontent with the Government at Nanking."[42]

According to Gale, *Time* had projected the generalissimo as the most powerful man in Asia and his kidnapper as a crazed dope fiend. *Time*'s reporters had not delved deeply in the real issue at the core of the friction. Moreover, they did not understand Chiang's agreement to a united front against the Japanese as a compromise executed in typically Chinese fashion.

Gale explained to supporters that *Time* had neither acknowledged the complexity of the problem, nor allowed American readers to understand the uniquely Chinese manner of its resolution.[43] Gale's experiences in China, her friendship with George Shepherd, and her relationship with her daughter Mary had allowed her to provide supporters with a different assessment of the Sian Incident. Able to perceive the grievances of Chiang's kidnappers as legitimate, Gale had sought to impart this knowledge to supporters in order to rectify what she rightfully perceived as the simplistic accounts offered to the American public by the media.

With the conclusion of the Sian Incident and Chiang's agreement to a Nationalist-Communist anti-Japanese united front, Gale was faced with the challenge of maintaining her optimism while explaining the less-than-promising developments in the Sino-Japanese War.

North China had been controlled by a semi-independent regime for over two years. However, when the first shot of the war was fired at Lukouch'iao on 7 July 1937, Chiang concluded that Japan wanted more direct control over China and that any Chinese reaction must be a strong one. Issuing the declaration that China must be prepared to sacrifice and "fight to the end," Chiang set the stage for total war and embarked upon the Shanghai campaign.

In August 1937, Chiang poured troops into the demilitarized zones around Shanghai (where his forces were superior in number to those of the Japanese) in violation of the 1932 Tangku agreement. Despite what began as vigorous pressure upon the Japanese, Chinese offensive capabilities were gradually worn down, and by 1 September, as the town of Wusung fell, the goal of the Chinese high command changed from offensive to positional warfare.[44]

Despite the bleak circumstances, Gale's assessment of China's position remained positive. Gale concluded that if the Chinese were sometimes "slow in their movements" it was not due to military inferiority but to the presence of a few disloyal, pro-Japanese elements within Nationalist ranks.[45] In September, despite the fall of Wusung, Gale described an angry Japanese military that could not budge the Chinese despite the presence of 120,000 troops.[46]

By October, troops from both sides poured into the seesaw battle which soon forced a Chinese retreat. However, rather than admit defeat, Gale focused upon the thrill of the entire nation at the bravery of the "doomed batallion" that had voluntarily withdrawn their lines.[47]

In November, Chiang moved the capital city from Nanking to Chungking, further emphasizing his resolve to fight, but that month the Nationalist military machine began to suffer a series of severe blows. By 9 November the Japanese Shanghai Expeditionary Force, with its six divisions and reinforcements totaling 200,000 men, forced the seventy-one division, 500,000-man Chinese force to retreat along the Nanking-Shanghai railway. Only shortly afterward, in December, came the well-known, brutal Japanese assault upon Nanking.[48]

At Shanghai, the Nationalist command had deployed about 60 percent of its forces and nearly all of its elite units.[49] By the end of 1937, the results had been disastrous: after a ninety-day struggle, the Japanese had stripped China of nearly all important centers of political power and industry.[50]

Gale interpreted this retreat as "part of some larger Chinese strategy."[51] Avoiding any admission of Chinese military inferiority or any hint that the retreat was anything but voluntary, Gale offered testimony to Chinese empowerment: she described the Chinese as heroic, their misgivings as isolated incidents caused by a few disloyal elements, and ultimately projected a humanitarian rationale for their defensive position. Gale argued that Chinese lines were withdrawn because Nationalist leaders believed it futile to sacrifice thousands of men when a slight retreat could save them.[52]

As one scholar has noted, however, the Shanghai Campaign may be viewed as the onset of a long attritional war in keeping with Chiang's belief that the best strategy against the Japanese was to "defend fixed positions to the last man." The loss of many battles and lives was necessary, probable, and intrinsic to Chiang's goal, not of saving lives but, of producing a war-weary Japan.[53]

While Chiang's goal did not change after January 1938, there was an important shift in emphasis: the depleted forces of the Shanghai campaign prompted him to advise his generals to harass the Japanese by conducting guerrilla warfare on all fronts.[54] With the start of 1938, the Chinese Nationalist government asserted its determination to switch to a posture of increased mobility, consolidating their forces in Wuhan, an important political and industrial center for central China.[55] At this stage of the war, Gale's admiration for Chinese Nationalist tactics was often combined with notice of Japanese military blunders and ineffectual occupation. These were emphasized in her correspondence to family and supporters from Nanchang, where the Gales relocated in response to the Nanchang General Hospital's requests for emergency medical assistance in November 1937.[56]

From Nanchang, Gale reported upon the infrequent Chinese successes which punctuated the eventual Japanese victory at Wuhan. As a prelude to their attack upon Wuhan, the Japanese had begun an offensive along the Peking-Pukow railway. By April, when one of Chiang's best generals lured their enemy into a trap killing approximately 30,000 Japanese, Gale reported, from her reading of Chinese newspapers, that Chinese guerrillas were cutting Japanese armies to pieces and that the Chinese had taken back places on three sides of Nanking and were pushing their forces inward. Gale noted happily that Japanese forces were evacuating, leaving no more than 2,000 in the Nanking area.[57]

Doubtlessly impressed with the Nationalists' April victory, which had led many in China to believe that with good leadership and weapons, the Chinese could hold their own, Gale described how Japanese plans backfired, benefiting their shrewd opponents.[58] Gale reported that combined Japanese ineptness and Chinese astuteness enabled the Chinese to obtain ammunition and food meant for the Japanese army.[59] By May 1938, Suchow had fallen, but Gale continued to make note of Japanese weakness.

By August 1938 Gale reported that the Japanese were no nearer Nanchang or Hankow than they had been in July, but the bigger, bleaker reality was that the Japanese had already assembled the planes, tanks, and artillery necessary for what would be the final assault on Wuhan. Gale acknowledged that the Japanese had succeeded in bombing Teh-An, where several refugees were trying to get to Nanchang, which had also been hit with a lot of bombs, but she considered these Japanese military victories insignificant.[60]

Not all women missionaries evinced Gale's optimism for China's military efforts. An alternative viewpoint of the Nanchang scene was described by Kiukiang, Kiangsi missionary Evaline Gaw. Secretary and treasurer of Kiukiang's Susan Toy Ensign Memorial Hospital, in her June 1938 correspondence to the Methodist Board:

> We feel that we have had quite a catastrophe . . . fall on Nanchang. The government has torn up the railroad between here and Kiukiang and are taking the rails and rolling stock farther west where they are building a road. We feel quite bereft. . . . The Chinese have held them quite steady for the past week or more, but it seems to me that the officials here have taken such a defeatist attitude. They fully expect the enemy to come. They do not seem to have faith that their troops can hold them.[61]

Unable to stand the unbearable summer heat of Nanchang, Gale left to spend two months at the popular summer resort at Kuling, beginning in the last week of June 1938.[62] While there, she once again took optimistic note of the Sino-Japanese power struggle.

At Kuling, Gale stayed in the Methodist valley, and she remarked that there were 538 people. Every entrance to the valley had a large painted American flag on it and very house had a small painted flag outside with a declaration from the American consul that the property was American. These precautions apparently protected both Chinese and foreigners from the Japanese. Gale noted that the "general opinion is that the enemy will not come up the hill." One Japanese officer declared that the Japanese had "no such intention—that their next objective was Nanchang."[63] Indeed, Gale noted that the foot of the mountain changed hands continuously during the summer of 1938 and that the Japanese would not dare bomb the area, filled with foreigners and Chinese. The Japanese were getting nowhere slowly in their quest for Nanchang, according to Gale. The Chinese were "putting up a stiff fight," and consequently, the Japanese were forced to send reinforcements many times. Gale was happy to report that outsiders observing the trenches noted the "splendid piece of work" done by the Chinese.[64]

By September 1938, Gale observed that the Japanese had left most of the Kuling area except the stations along the railroad to Nanchang and that they had had to give up one of their four roads to Hankow. It was "inferred," Gale noted, that they had squandered too many men and spent too much money, having dropped bombs "like water and accomplished very little."[65] Yet, despite the optimism Gale felt toward China, by October, Chiang Kai-shek lost de facto control over eastern China, the country's most fertile farmland, and an area rich in commercial and industrial wealth.[66]

Gale's summer of 1939 correspondence contained explicit evidence of Chinese advantages, and it represented many of the themes Gale had reiterated since 1931. It was relayed, via a United States-bound Presbyterian family, to Gale's son Lester who mimeographed copies for all mission field supporters. Gale's account was tempered by fear, as tension had been heightened due to a recent poisoning in the Japanese consulate; however, it presented an especially rosy picture. She noted that Chinese guerrillas, numbering hundreds of thousands, had succeeded in accosting the enemy all over the "so called" occupied territory. The Japanese could not leave the cities, and they did not dare go off the main streets.[67] She described her 1938 Christmas: with a group of thirty British, American and Swedish people, she had come down the mountain from Kuling, escorted by Nationalists, British officers, and Americans. Upon reaching Japanese-occupied territory, Gale reiterated impressions formulated during the first phase of the Japanese invasion, depicting the bravery and humanity of the Chinese.[68]

> The Japanese have the large cities pretty well garrisoned and a thin line of sentry "pill-boxes" as far apart as telephone poles along the railroad. But a friend who recently made a trip . . . says the enemy are jittery. He says he believes the Chinese could take the railroads back at any time they wish. Why do they not do so? Because if anything happens along the line the nearest village or town is blamed and every man and woman and child is put to death.[69]

Gale had accurately described Japanese occupation of China but had exaggerated accounts of Chinese humanity. Chinese military power was not only tempered by humanity but also aided by a flimsy Japanese occupation. Gale explained her agreement with a Catholic Bishop who compared the Japanese to amoebas swimming in a basin of water. Tens of thousands of Chinese in the "occupied areas do not know what a Japanese look like. That can be said of villages very near here." The hold of the Japanese was a "vague one," conditioned upon the existence of large guns, gunboats and airplanes. In this sense, concluded Gale, the term "occupied territory" was truly a "misnomer."[70]

Gale's correspondence emphasized that the Japanese exaggerated reports of military victory. For example, in September 1937, during Chiang's Shanghai Campaign, Gale compared Japanese reports that twenty-three Chinese planes had gone down in Nanking with Chinese government statements that only twelve planes had gone up and only a few had been hit.[71]

In February 1938, Gale noted that the Japanese had reported the downing of seven planes, when in actuality, there had only been one.[72] One month later, she admitted that six of "our" (Chinese) planes had been brought down in the February attack, but emphasized that eight Japanese planes were downed. In addition, Gale refuted Japanese boasts that they had "brought order to the city of Nanking." She forwarded a translated Japanese article describing Japanese activities in Nanking along with one Nanking missionary's assessment, so that readers could contrast both. The Japanese described the excellent treatment, including medical, that they offered to the Chinese in Nanking. The missionary described how the Japanese terrorized Chinese women. Indeed, the missionary described how their collective horror at Japanese atrocities led missionaries to temporarily put safety before morality and set up designated "Red Light" districts for the Japanese.[73]

Another important aspect of Gale's portrayal of the Sino-Japanese war was her insistence that Chinese strength and ability were inversely proportional to Japanese aggression. Gale reiterated an account of WFMS missionary Katherine Boeye's experiences during the bombing of Chungking in a 1939 letter to her supporters at the Simpson Church. The Japanese had been inhumanely cruel, dropping 109 bombs, some incendiary, in about five seconds in the midst of the most congested residential and business section, just as many of the city's populace were finishing the day's work. The estimated number of casualties was 5,000, and there could be no mistaking Japanese intentions to hurt civilians and thus break the morale of the Chinese: there had not been a military post nor a government building in the entire area.[74]

Despite the severity of the losses, Gale emphasized that the attack had the effect of strengthening Chinese resolve to fight to the end. Gale explained to readers that Chinese optimism grew out of the belief that

"God did give them this country . . . ," thus, while bombings were meant to demoralize, they had the opposite effect.[75]

Japanese military atrocities horrified Gale, and like all missionaries, she reiterated her abhorrence to supporters. However, her admiration for Asian cultures led her to make a clear differentiation between the Japanese military and its people. She viewed the Japanese as modern and, like the Chinese, appreciative of beauty and aesthetically refined. Gale believed that Japanese civilians, kept in the dark by the lies of militarists, were blind to the thievery motivating the aggression against China.[76] Thus, the Japanese enemy was a satanic force, separate from the whole of the Japanese nation from which it originated.

Noting the insignia on their planes, Gale called the Japanese military "Red devils;"[77] however, she viewed individual Japanese, businessmen and many soldiers as fine human beings, wishing only to "save their face" before it was too late. While some soldiers committed horrific acts, many Japanese soldiers viewed their present situation with "dread." Japanese business people were so "taxed by their own government and their businesses" had become so small that they only wished to return to Japan.[78] Gale believed that there was "hope for Japan . . . if only there was some way to get the truth" to the Japanese people. She asked: "Why should a few militarists ruin a fine nation?"[79] Gale implied that if the Japanese people could take back control of their government, there was still hope for their nation's redemption.

In Gale's mind, Christianity was a bond more powerful than the effects of the Sino-Japanese War, and it played a key part in her belief in the potential for goodness in all people and eventual peace. Gale told the story of one Christian Japanese captain, given the order to execute thirty Chinese soldiers and a pastor. During the final moments the group began to sing a Christian hymn. Upon hearing their voices, the captain froze in his tracks, remembering his own early Christian background. He then countermanded the order of execution, freeing the group.[80]

Gale's Christian interpretation of the war helps one understand her impressions of its progress.[81] In Shanghai, during both 1932 and 1937, the forces of God and the devil were clearly drawn: the latter was a callous Japanese military. The former were Chiang's forces, whose Christian moral courage would lead them to beat the odds.

By 1939, Gale's assertion of China's unity under Chiang was correct: the entire nation, Communists included, were behind the generalissimo in his resolve to fight the Japanese.[82] Moreover, Gale projected a Chinese people, unified in their quest for national self-determination, as akin to Americans in their earlier struggle against the British.

As has been noted, Gale was like many missionaries in her tendency to project an affinity, beginning with the birth of the Chinese Republic in 1911, between Chinese and Americans. Comparing the Sino-Japanese War to the American Revolution, Gale declared Chiang Kai-shek to be China's George Washington. Referring to the few pro-Japanese elements still remaining, Gale explained that there were traitors in China, as there had been during the American war for independence. In the end, Gale predicted that since God had brought the right side to victory after the American Revolution, he would do so for China.[83]

Sino-American affinity was relegated to the personal as well as national level, as foreigners and Chinese experienced the exigent circumstances of war, aware of sharing an uncertain destiny. Gale described Nanchang's "people . . . on the go with their bundles of clothes . . . literally millions of people going somewhere to try to get away from the enemy."[84] In August 1938, Gale noted that in wartime all people, including herself and her husband, were in danger of being separated from their loved ones and could "expect anything." Gale said goodbye to her husband in late 1937, when he went off on a special assignment to the Wuhu Hospital, and while she thought their separation would only last a few weeks, it would last nine months.[85] The Chinese passing through Kuling had experienced the same plight as the Gales. There was a constant feeding of refugees, with a daily average of from 500 to 700. According to Gale, these were "patient" people, caught between the firing lines.[86] Indeed, Gale suggested to supporters that she considered herself one of a "huge multitude" of people (Chinese and foreign) who were separated from "homes, friends or relatives."[87]

Those who took refuge with Gale in the mountain resort at Kuling, a total of 6,880 registered people (180 foreigners), awakened daily to the sound of machine guns. Gale observed that, despite assurances that the Japanese only wanted Nanchang, everyone—Americans, foreigners and Chinese—shared a common terror that one day the Japanese would climb the hill and slaughter them as they had "raped Nanking."[88] Thus, Gale projected Chinese and foreigners alike in their wartime struggles. Doubtlessly, mission field supporters understood this when Gale concluded her accounts with the comment: "our sufferings mingle with theirs."[89]

To Gale's long history of projecting professional and personal success to supporters, she could add the Sino-Japanese war, an arduous test of her own competency. Despite the inevitable frustrations she had likely encountered, Gale's accounts of medical successes in Nanchang led supporters to believe that she met her challenges with flying colors. She arrived in Nanchang in November 1937 to find that wounded soldiers not only filled the 160-bed Nanchang Hospital, but an additional 100 beds in the Nanchang boys' school. Gale was assigned to the most seriously wounded in the upper floor of the boys' school. One month later Gale told Simpson Church supporters that she had sole charge of the treatment of 240 severely wounded soldiers, as well as the 100 boys in the Nanchang boys' school.[90]

At Nanchang, Gale came to face to face with the ravages of Japanese aggression: "It makes one's heart ache to see these blasted arms and legs when the cause is the desire" of the Japanese to steal China's land, she noted to her son Frank.[91] Gale told Simpson Church supporters of working alone for two weeks, except for the help of some Chinese girls with first aid training: "I dressed wrecked arms, legs and hands" from morning until late afernoon, as the wounded soldiers never stopped coming.[92]

Gale her juxtaposed her expertise to the inadequacies of a male doctor without revealing his national identity. For one month a group of soldiers had had only Gale do their dressings; however, one day, feeling ill, she had taken to her bed. The following day Gale learned that her soldiers had been in great distress: the physician who had taken over her duties had not been as competent as she, and the soldiers feared her departure was permanent. The soldiers had protested vehemently. While Gale had empathized with the physical discomforts of the men, she had been glad to be appreciated.[93]

Pride in her professional accomplishments reflected Gale's belief in an order where competence was a source of individual power regardless of gender or race. Gale projected the idea that she was not only gentler, (perhaps by virtue of her gender) but more competent than the male physician. This same belief had precluded Gale from giving most of her emphasis to the crippling effects of war on individual Chinese. Instead, Gale preferred to emphasize that there were no obstacles large enough, whether they be gender, race prejudice or military devastation, to challenge the power of Christianity.

In May 1938, when Gale was preparing to give a church sermon, she answered a question that many Chinese Christians repeatedly posed to her: "Why doesn't God do something?" Gale was certain that she was right when she explained: "God is perfect wisdom and when he gave man free will he reserved the final results to be in his own power. The world killed Christ but the final result was with God—the Resurrection. China may be crucified but God's final purpose cannot be changed." Ultimately, dominion lay with God who would see to it that the Japanese, like all aggressor nations, would pay for their excesses.[94]

While the Sino-Japanese War brought tragic and needless loss of lives and property, Gale was like many missionaries in her belief that it also did much to strengthen the cause of Christianity. Thus, while she did not believe China would "go Christian as a result of the war," she did feel that "Christianity has received what may prove its greatest impetus in Chinese history."[95]

These beliefs were emphasized by Gale while she was on furlough in the United States from 1940 to 1941. During this critical period leading to the formal Sino-American alliance of World War II, Gale spoke to many other religious and other groups, besides her former classmates, friends and local residents at Colorado College. In Illinois Gale gave over forty talks in two weeks. In Chicago, for example, she spoke to twelve churches and eleven school groups, including one group of 300 high school students. While Gale's private letters do not reveal the content of her talks, they record the presence of curious audience members who asked many questions about China.[96] As noted by *The Tiger*, Gale's talks reflected her optimism in China's ability to win the war against her aggressor. As indicated by Gale's correspondence to friends and supporters, the home field had been cognizant of this theme during the years leading up to Japanese attack upon Pearl Harbor in December of 1941.

Gale's perceptions and portayal of the Sino-Japanese war offer an alternate interpretation to most scholars' definitions of the Sino-American friendship. Most often scholars describe this friendship as predicated upon the belief in the American public's desire to see China in their own nation's image. This wish is perceived by scholars as intertwined with, and rationalized by, a belief in the hierarchical classification of race and gender. In other words, scholars believe the special Sino-American friendship did much to strengthen conceptions of both the dominance of men in the domestic realm and the United States in the international arena.[97]

Scholars have labeled American images of China "female,"[98] but by correlating female concerns to empowerment by piety, a vehicle for subverting male dominance, Gale redefined the meaning of the term "female." During her Nanking years, she gave supporters' evidence that Chinese Nationalists had accepted Protestantism and the need to attend to social issues, particularly public health. In addition, Gale argued that the Nationalists gave evidence of supporting a public role for Chinese women. Gale told supporters that Nationalist leaders believed Chinese women should have an important role in the reconstruction of China. Thus, while Gale depicted China's government as having promoted humanistic values she intertwined this with the message that Chinese women were accepted as men's equals and that the Chinese nation was a modern, progressive one, based upon the status of its women.

Belief in empowerment through piety led Gale to define "female," when empowered by piety, as strong, rather than weak. China had supported programs and ideas which, in the United States were deemed inferior by those mainstream Americans who shunned such traditionally female values as "social concern" and valued scientific medicine over the more humanistic role of the physician. From Gale's and women supporters' perspectives, these values represented a vehicle for empowerment for women, and in China, they had been a vehicle for empowerment for Gale, whose self-representations suggested power, autonomy and success.

Since Gale viewed the Chinese nation as empowered through piety, the Japanese attack did not represent male strength (Japanese) and female weakness (Chinese) but male power abuse and women's empowerment-through-piety. Gale depicted Chiang as the assured victor in the Sino-Japanese war, and proof of his Christianity was his presumably humane military strategy.

While China lacked the military preparedness of the Japanese, depicted by most observers in typically male images, Gale did not suggest that the war reflected China's need for parenting. Rather, Gale's portrayals of heroic Chinese soldiers, the Cantonese army, Chiang's astute military strategies and his humanitarian motivations, suggest that China was not child-like, in her need for support, but strong in her ability to combat the "Satanic" Japanese military.[99] While Gale may have privately believed in Western superiority, she encouraged Americans to support the Chinese, not because the Chinese were weak, but because she believed it each individual's duty to maintain a world order based upon cooperation, a typically female concern.

Gale's images of China were especially important because they went beyond the simplistic accounts of the media. She shared with supporters her own wish to learn the truth about political developments in China, and her willingness to rely upon Chinese, as well as Westerners to do so. The influence of the Chinese in her life, supporters of Feng Yu-hsiang, the Chinese poor, and her daughter Mary, prompted Gale to suggest, during the time of the Sian Incident, that even a Christian Chinese leader such as Chiang could be wrong, and that the anti-Christian Communists could be correct. However, Gale's respect for Chinese know-how superseded any admission of Christian Chinese weakness: it demonstrated to American supporters that an empowered American woman felt that she had much to learn from the Chinese.

While Chiang had established such reforms as the 1932 Civil Code banning arranged marriages and giving sons and daughters equal inheritance rights, by the late 1920s, Chinese feminists and some missionaries recognized that the New Life movement had been based upon profoundly conservative perceptions of women and men. Perhaps it was because of her affinity with George Shepherd, or her insistence that Chiang was a Christian, that Gale had overstated Nationalists' espousal of women Protestant's conception of social concern, and obscured the actual setbacks experienced by Chinese women as a result of Chiang's oppressive policies.[100] Moreover, as has been shown, Gale naively ignored the inhumanity of Chiang's military maneuvers. With all of its inaccuracies and contradictions, Gale's message to women supporters was pleasing: a military victory for China was a victory for Christianity and for the power of values traditionally associated with them.

8

Chadwick Memorial Hospital, Tzechung

ARRIVING IN HONG KONG ON 20 NOVEMBER 1941, GALE FACED HER first of a series of wartime challenges.[1] While Reverend Gale was told that he could disembark from the *President Harrison*, she was forced to remain on board until she agreed to sign a $250 bond with a promise to leave within two weeks.[2] The Gales would leave the city separately: while they agreed to eventually meet in West China, where Dr. Gale would begin medical work, Rev. Gale set off to see his Chinese pastors and get some family possessions from the Gales' Nanking home.[3]

Reverend Gale's passage through Shanghai coincided with the 7 December 1941 bombing of Pearl Harbor, the United States declaration of war against Japan, and the Japanese sequestration of foreigners in occupied territory in eastern China. Reverend Gale's isolation by the Japanese was followed by four years in a Japanese internment camp in Shanghai and one year as superintendent of the Nanchang General Hospital: a five year separation from his wife.[4]

Departing from Hong Kong on the last plane leaving that city, Gale was delayed for one month in Chungking, finally arriving in Tzechung, West China in January 1942.[5] She was sixty-three years old, an age when many women retired to a life of leisure, but Gale's arrival to Tzechung, and her work at Chadwick Memorial hospital, marked the onset of five productive years as hospital administrator.

The Tzechung hospital had undergone some difficulties immediately prior to Gale's arrival.[6] For two years, the thirty-year-old hospital had been under the administration of WFMS missionary, Dr. Ruth Hemenway.[7] Soon after Gale's arrival, she observed that the hospital had suffered from a bad reputation caused by Hemenway's difficulties in dealing with those Tzechung people within "the staff and with the citizens who had folks in the hospital." In her correspondence to the Methodist Board, Gale reiterated the sentiment of many Chinese and Westerners who felt that the hospital was still suffering from "some of the animosity caused at" the time Hemenway was in charge.[8] Hemenway had experienced frustration with the Tzechung mayor and his entourage, whom she disparagingly referred to as "ignorant practitioners of Chinese-style medicine." Hemenway reported that by January 1940 the mayor had established a small hospital at the gate of the city of about 80,000. To Hemenway's apparent dismay, when gauze and drugs arrived from any outside organization, the mayor would steer these goods toward his own hospital, rather than that of Hemenway. In retaliation, Hemenway set out to prove that her hospital workers were better skilled than the mayor's in their ability to treat bombing victims. The confrontation that ensued made the mayor's hospital appear inadequate, led to his loss of face and subsequently the mayor and the city's populace would become hostile toward Hemenway and the hospital.[9]

Knowledge of its bad reputation had motivated Gale to want to promote good feeling for her hospital among Tzechung residents. Gale's desire was to create a hospital that the entire populace could be proud of—a first-rate, modern institution. This was not an easy task, considering the extent of Gale's responsibilities as a physician in Tzechung.

Gale described her program of medical duties as "very heavy." She held a daily clinic at the Tzechung girls' school and a women's clinic three times a week. At the hospital, she was in charge of religious work and supervised the nurses and the coolies who did the hospital cleaning. In addition, Gale was expected to account for the hospital furniture, instruments, drugs and linens.[10] Gale's goal of creating a first-rate institution was also hampered, not only by a hectic schedule, but also by the condition of the hospital in early 1942.

The thirty-bed Chadwick Memorial hospital was built from local sandstone and made a "very fine appearance,"[11] but its attractive exterior belied its numerous problems. The hospital had a large deficit and, consequently, was poorly equipped. Chadwick Memorial's lack of funds resulted in even more work for Gale: in addition to her medical duties, Gale found herself unwillingly thrust into the position of hospital administrator and treasurer. As she recognized, the most difficult aspect of her new responsibilities would be, not only keeping the records, but also finding funds to cover the existing deficit.[12]

Gale found that the most pressing problem faced by the hospital was its shortage of nurses: most were attracted to work for the higher paying hospitals such as those in the larger West China cities of Chengtu and Chungking.[13] Moreover, the shortage had a serious effect on staff physicians. Chadwick Hospital's nursing shortage dictated that all doctors take on the responsibility of preparing their own instruments and linens for major operations, as well as providing patient medications. In addition to her other duties, for example, Gale was in charge of bathing and caring for two tiny babies and three children ill with dysentery, duties normally executed by nurses.

In part, Gale's problem was resolved by securing supporter promises to contribute enough to double four nurses' salaries to match the money paid by large hospitals.[14] However, in keeping with her past experience as a hospital administrator, Gale understood that attracting nurses to her hospital required more than just higher salaries. She believed that the "greatest need" was for adequate living quarters where nurses could have sufficient space to be comfortable and entertain their friends.

Acting upon her past experiences in Tunki and at the Nanchang General Hospital, Gale took the initiative of designing the ideal living environment she envisioned. She drew a sketch of two floors of housing accommodations: the first floor would contain the nurses' apartments and the second floor, a living room and additional small rooms. As in the past, Gale reported that those around her were responsive to her ideas. Gale told the Methodist Board that her sketch was well received at the first hospital board meeting, soon after her arrival. One of the doctors appointed an architect to draw Gale's plans, and soon afterward, estimates were obtained. Gale reiterated this story to supporters, advertising her request for funds to support her plan in Methodist Advocates throughout the United States, and the *World Outlook*.[15]

Adding to supporters' knowledge of Gale's plans to raise nurses' salaries and renovate their living quarters, were West China medical missionary, Dr. Howard Liljestrand's accounts of Gale's innovative activities. Liljestrand confirmed Gale's ability to take strong action against the nursing shortage: in September 1942, he told supporters that Gale was doing "heroic service" in starting a nursing school.[16] Gale soon reported that despite some early problems, the school was well established.[17] This correspondence from the mission field, and advertisements directed to contributors helped enhance Gale's credibility as an assertive, creative doctor, capable of shaping conditions around her despite the hardships of war, thus suggesting that women doctors were men's equals in administrative matters.

In keeping with women medical missionaries' proclivity to concern themselves with the whole patient, apart from the disease, Gale concerned herself with the more humanistic endeavors that would appeal to many American women contributors: Gale reported that she worked to improve the lot of Tzechung's poor. She explained that since her arrival in January of 1942, "it has been on my heart to see if some way could not be found to start a half-time day school." She was in Tzechung less than one year when she achieved her goal. By 10 September 1942 Gale would find a teacher, hold registration, and one week later, begin a half-time day school for poor Chinese children in the area.[18]

Creating the small school was one aspect of her efforts for Tzechung's poorer residents: since her arrival to Tzechung, Gale had reported her distress at the low numbers of poor who could take advantage of the hospital's services. With its economic difficulties, the hospital initially had no funds for poor Chinese in need of medical treatment. Gale's first step was to ask supporters to send contributions so that the hospital could set up a "poor fund."[19]

The eventual success of this fund was made possible by Chinese Bishop Chen, whom Gale described to supporters as "the hope of China."[20] She had confided in Chen, a pastor and former leader of the National Christian Council, regarding her wish for the fund, and he had responded by requesting the Methodist Committee on Overseas Relief to send enough monies to set up a poor fund for the Chadwick Memorial Hospital.[21]

Supporters' willingness to continue contributing to the poor fund, either directly to Gale or through the Methodist Committee on Overseas Relief, was doubtlessly stimulated by Gale's projection of Chinese recipients as what Gale designated as the "deserving poor." Harkening back to nineteenth-century Victorian values of self-sufficiency, Gale described worthy, honorable, hard-working Chinese people for whom Gale worked as their doctor and social worker. In this capacity, she depicted each patient's medical needs as interwoven with his life circumstances. In each case, Gale described poor fund beneficiaries as individuals and families who sought work, but were unable to do so because of incapacitating physical ailments.[22] Gale described some cases in great detail in order to encourage supporters to feel that they were as important as she in implementing her goals, and that it was a joint effort, a reciprocal relationship between supporter and missionary. Gale told supporters: "I know you will want to hear of some of these interesting cases for it is your working together with us that has made this possible."[23]

Gale cured the family of one self-supporting farmer who had been emaciated by hook and long worm. She used the hospital's poor fund to cure the father and children, then proceeded to help the family begin a business making straw sandals.[24]

Gale was careful to explain that "present circumstances" forced the Chinese to consider certain options merely to survive. She believed beggars "deserving" because they either could not, or simply had not been given the opportunity to work. Two little boys, reduced to begging, were given physical and economic help at the hospital. One boy had been forced to beg when his family became desperately hungry due to the increasingly high price of food. Despite the painful hernia he developed, he had had the intelligence and perseverance to walk to the Chadwick hospital. While there, an operation cured him and he found a home with a relative.[25]

Another little boy was picked up from the side of the road and brought to the hospital by a passerby. Surrendering to his pain with endless moaning, and unwilling to speak to anyone, the little boy initially appeared beyond hope. With the nurses' persistent feedings and visits by Methodist schoolgirls on Sunday, however, Gale reported that the little boy soon turned into a smiling, talkative child who followed doctors around, anxious to help. Gale and her hospital staff worked to help the boy find an apprenticeship to learn a trade to support himself.[26]

Gale was able to treat a farmer gored by a water buffalo. The family was determined to pay for treatment, but ran out of money after the man's first week at the hospital. Since this was far short of the time needed for successful recovery, Gale told supporters that their poor fund was responsible for supplying the cost of the additional time necessary for the farmer's survival.[27]

Gale described the Chinese poor as individuals who were either already strong and independent or strove to be so. There were blind men, eager to have their sight restored so that they would not need to be led. A Chinese doctor at Chadwick Hospital successfully treated three for trachoma. One boatman with an infected arm was initially too proud to solicit help on his own, but eventually was treated by the hospital. A seventeen-year-old leper was no victim, according to Gale, but a man of strong character, whose disease was not too far advanced for cure.

Eager to present a positive picture, Gale did not reiterate the stories of those whose lives were lost due to insufficient resources. Rather, supporters were told only of all the worthy and admirable individuals who were cured by their contributions.[28]

After two years, Gale told supporters that the hospital took in eighty-two "poor folk who otherwise could not have had any medical care" and provided free medicine to 2,311 at the hospital clinic.[29] By January 1947, five years after her arrival, Gale was happy to report that over 13 percent of the patients in the hospital and clinic were treated without charge due to supporters' contributions to the poor fund.[30]

While Gale was eager to share her successes with the home field, it is likely that these happy anecdotes were rendered even more significant by the manner in which she chose to explain the problems she faced. For example, Gale initially considered herself a neophyte in the area of accounting,[31] and indeed, at the close of her first year in Tzechung, she told supporters that the hospital still had a small deficit.[32] While Gale did not describe a desperate situation to supporters, privately, she admitted that during her first year she had struggled with a hospital deficit and a coworker who confessed to stealing from the hospital. Indeed, in a 1943 letter to the Methodist Board, Gale had admitted that "this has been about the most upsetting year of my missionary experience."[33] In short, Gale would present obstacles in a manner which would enhance, rather than dampen, supporters' enthusiasm, and she would consciously hide her despair in order to maintain supporters' optimism.

In Tunki, Gale had infused excitement into her appeals for monies by making supporters feel as though they had had an important hand in helping her create a hospital where none existed. Likewise, her letters from Tzechung were designed to make supporters feel as though the obstacles and victories Gale experienced during wartime were partially a result of their doings. For example, after two years of describing the "miserable little oil wicks we have to use," Gale told supporters that finally "we have electric lights!"[34]

In 1944, Gale described the hospital's portable electric plant:

> Most of you remember that we were already wired for electricity, but we have not been able to use the large plant on account of the expense. This one is small and cheaply run.[35]

Thus, Gale was able to assure supporters that the hospital was functioning cost-effectively, while simultaneously suggesting that it could take full advantage of its electricity with future supporter contributions for a larger plant. While Gale's descriptions were meant to suggest that supporters look toward the future, they also harkened back to the past, drawing upon the four decades of correspondence Gale had shared with them. She asked supporters to recall their assistance to her in Tunki:

> I wonder how many of you dear folks can remember that many years ago— nearly twenty . . . I wrote you about my ambition to "raise the roof." That was far away off in another province and was an attempt to make a little house over into a hospital. . . . I remember how wonderfully you responded and the deed was done. Recently my mind has been running along the same lines.[36]

Gale presented her problem, the lack of room for new patients, as a consequence of the hospital's success. She asked supporters to contribute once again to "raising the roof," as "we are growing out of our quarters." As Gale noted, an important reason for the hospital's increasing popularity was the government's decision that it would be "one of the hospitals that are to care for those sick in government service."[37]

Gale's intention to make supporters feel directly responsible for solving her problems led the home field to contribute to American relief organizations. Gale was one of many missionaries who helped generate the large sums of money raised by the American Red Cross (ARC) for China during the 1940s. By the end of 1941, for example, the ARC provided $2,936,124.00 in relief to China. While clothing represented the largest Red Cross relief item, medical and sanitary supplies, food, blankets, bedding and cash were large-scale ARC efforts for which China was a leading recipient.[38] Gale's messages to supporters represented one factor that helped make it possible for the ARC to raise these large sums.

Gale told supporters that despite the prohibitive cost of drugs, instruments, a blood pressure apparatus, cotton, gauze and unbleached muslin, supporter contributions to the American Red Cross, the International Relief Committee and the Methodist Relief Committee, insured her continued acquisition of these items.[39] Gale described her initial desperation, each time supplies would run ominously low, and subsequent joy when her needs were met by the organizations to which supporters contributed.

For example, in 1944 the superintendent of nurses had just given Gale a report indicating that a shortage in cloth would mean patients' pillows would not have cases. Shortly afterward a bale of cloth arrived from the Red Cross. Gale described how the cloth would provide, not only pillow cases, but sheets, bedspreads and even nurses' uniforms. Many times, poor, nearly blind patients arrived and Gale told supporters' that their contributions to relief organizations relieved "the cause" and brought "permanent cure," by enabling her to perform sight-saving eye operations.[40]

Gale reported that had it not been for supporter contributions to the International Relief Committee, the American Red Cross and the Methodist Relief Funds, the hospital would "have been in desperate straits to provide even rice for our doctors, and nurses and servants, not to mention the poor patients." Instead, Gale reported that "we have had an outstanding year," with "more patients in the hospital and more at the clinics." An old ward was "recovered," and wooden beds, chairs and tables were made. The hospital's sandstone exterior was given a fresh coat of paint, and the walls, halls, and rooms were restored.[41]

Gale depicted her hospital as an institution that could bond Chinese and Americans in the common goal of helping the needy. Gale told supporters that a poor mother brought her son, ill with diphteria, to her clinic. The necessary treatment would require two injections costing $15,000 each. Another Chinese patient in the hospital, a ship owner, offered to pay for part of the serum. Gale explained that supporter funds provided the remaining sum necessary: "So you and this neighbor were both Good Samaritans," Gale told supporters.[42]

Those supporters who were more interested in the Chinese upper-classes than work for the needy doubtlessly found stimulating material in Gale's depictions of the Chinese gentry and officials' growing admiration for her hospital. As has been stated, Gale hoped that all Tzechung citizens would eventually come to feel that the Chadwick Memorial Hospital was their own, and that they would trust it to treat their illnesses and that of family and friends. One male doctor suggested to Gale that a "sudden revival" would help the popularity of the hospital. While Gale would have welcomed a revival, she perceived the popularity of the Chadwick Memorial Hospital as stemming from "gradual acceptance . . . bit by bit and day by day, one patient" passing "the word on to another."[43]

Supporter contributions were a great factor in her ability to win the approval of the conservative Tzechung populace. Gale admitted that, upon arrival, people had not always agreed to medical treatment. Indeed, in January 1942, they had been antagonistic.[44] Had she not had sufficient funds to paint, repair, and clean, the conservative Tzechung gentry would not have perceived the hospital as "up and coming."[45] The gentry's approval, in turn, influenced the attitude of others toward the hospital.

Inadvertently evincing her feelings of superiority, Gale professed the belief that some of her hospital's status had come from her willingness to demand respect from Chinese in positions of power. For example, in 1944, an officer struck a Chinese doctor because his soldier was dying in the hospital. Gale angrily approached the official in charge, demanding an apology. While the officer threatened to send no more soldiers to the hospital, the opposite occurred. Gale soon found that she had more officers, soldiers, and conscripts than ever before and attributed this to the courage she displayed in standing up to the officer.[46]

Gale believed that her perseverance was another reason for the high status of her hospital. Gale obtained an x-ray machine, which increased the credibility of the hospital, with a persistent two-year letter writing campaign to two other missionaries. As noted, in 1944, she described to supporters how she had obtained a portable electric plant for the hospital and how she had looked forward to being able to use this electricity for an x-ray machine so that patients would not have to be sent to the Chengtu hospital for x-rays.[47] Gale had written many letters requesting that when United States forces left, she might have access to various supplies that they were leaving behind. When they finally left, Gale acquired the complete x-ray machine, fluoroscope and a generator which furnished electric lights for the hospital for the bargain price of $3,300.[48]

Gale described the way in which her business acumen allowed her to furnish a hospital with modern equipment. She began to decrease her hospital's deficit after only six months in Tzechung by establishing clinics for wealthy business people. She had made an agreement to provide nearby alcohol factories with clinics three times a week for a fee of $2,000 per month. These fees solidified her ties with Tzechung's business sector, and helped compensate for the exorbitant cost of patients' food and supplies.[49]

Perhaps because of Gale's knowledge of the past difficulties that Dr. Hemenway had faced, in her letters to supporters, she emphasized her respect for the Tzechung gentry and her friendship with the district magistrate and the mayor.[50] In 1945, Gale noted with surprise and pleasure that a group of aristocratic young men from a nearby government school asked to use her hospital as a background for their class picture, and they insisted that the name of the hospital be visible.[51] In a personal letter to Frank Cartwright in 1947, Gale reported victory: the entire community was "changed toward the hospital. They are proud of it, so I think there will be nothing but progress in the future. They are sold on Western Medicine."[52]

What Gale considered the most significant proof of her success in Tzechung were the increasing numbers of individuals willing to be treated by the hospital for their ailments. In describing this growing phenomenon, Gale was careful to provide a positive picture. Just three months after arrival, Gale had reported to supporters that she was very busy providing daily treatment to 50 to 80 of the 380 Tzechung schoolgirls. There was an abundance of trachoma, "itch," athlete's foot, ringworm and other skin disorders. She noted that the girls had been "so willing to come for treatment," an encouraging sign, considering that "this is said to be a very conservative city and foreign medicine has been slow in gaining acceptance here."[53]

Similarly, in a 1942 letter to supporters, the director of the West China Conference Medical Work noted Gale's enormous victory in being able to treat 70 percent of the trachoma cases in the Tzechung school for girls while simultaneously succeeding in the financial phase of the hospital work, as treasurer and accountant and performing "considerable clinical and obstetrical work."[54] Despite these positive accounts, Gale remembered her first months in Tzechung much less optimistically a few years later.[55]

In 1944, Gale admitted to supporters that when she had first arrived in Tzechung, the parents at the Tzechung Girls' School had not been willing to utilize her medical services. Gale recalled that this attitude also prevailed among the students, parents and the teachers. Gale's response was to "spend much time at the clinic trying to win them to see the advantages of our kind of treatment." She felt that by 1944 she had succeeded. Gale noted that during the past year, many of the girls were willing and ready to go to the hospital. One girl who had been very resistant to Gale had become her greatest helper, "bringing others along with her." The school's principal had become a patient in the hospital.[56]

In 1945, Gale reported that her progress continued. That year the girls developed ringworm, athlete's foot, boils and trachoma and many sought treatment in Gale's clinic. In May of that year there came a greater test of Gale's medical skills: a flu epidemic. Three years earlier the parents took their daughters home, but now Gale noted that their experience with Western medicine had prompted them to place their daughters' lives in her hands. Gale's response was to spring into immediate and decisive action: she turned one building of the school into a second hospital, provided the girls with twenty-four hour nursing service and closed all classes for a week. Gale reported that she was successful in treating the girls.[57]

Gale told supporters that Americans and Chinese appreciated her hospital. In 1944, for example, Gale noted that one doctor who was in charge of International Relief work visited the Chadwick Memorial hospital twice, expressing his admiration for Gale's ability to administer despite the difficult wartime conditions. She noted that the difficulties did not seem so great "after we knew that folks felt we were mastering them."[58]

In 1945, Gale reported that a United States officer, a friend of Gale's American coworker, visited the hospital after two years of living in huts, sleeping on army cots and eating at a soldiers' mess. Inadvertently disparaging her host country, while simultaneously elevating the notion of female competency in medical administration, Gale boasted to supporters that the officer was surprised to find such a fine hospital "over here in China."[59]

A former missionary in California told Gale that her hospital was reportedly the best one in the province and the only one of its size in West China with an x-ray machine. As Gale reminded readers: the hospital had gone from debt and bad condition to a surplus in monies, coal and rice. Moreover, its building structure had been repaired and an annex completed.[60]

After two years of providing funds for the hospital poor and reporting that a surplus grew in the hospital budget, Gale reveled in the uniqueness of her talents, noting that "I hear so many of the hospitals" are in a "hole."[61] Gale's quarterly letters supported her accounts of success with statistics.

In a 1946 letter to supporters, Gale recapitulated the results of four successful years. Since 1942, the numbers of hospital inpatients had nearly doubled, from 478 to 967. Outpatients in the clinic had more than tripled, from 5,248 to 16,136, and obstetrical cases multiplied over five-fold, from 10 to 55. The number of operations performed went from 104 to 262 and laboratory tests rose from 832 to 3,764. In 1942 the hospital had had no pharmacy, but five years later, a professional pharmacist filled 8,286 prescriptions.[62] Moreover, by the beginning of 1946, the hospital had expanded from 30 to 65 beds.[63]

Gale told supporters that she had created the first-rate hospital she had dreamed of, complete with electric lights and an x-ray machine, despite the hardships of world war and China's economic and political crises. She proclaimed to have won the admiration of the entire Tzechung populace, who had come to perceive the Chadwick Hospital an effective, modern facility.

Alongside Gale's carefully detailed accounts of successful medical work, and supporters' contributions to it, were her descriptions of the significance of the American military presence in China. Written to inspire pride among the home field, Gale's wartime depictions were written to help stimulate American support for the Sino-American alliance.

Five months after her arrival in 1942, Gale described how the Tzechung populace lived in dugouts the year before, comparing it to the present peaceful state, which was due to Allied bomber planes. When she heard the passing Royal Air Force planes, she experienced a "restful" feeling in her "heart." As she told supporters, her peace of mind was owed to the certainty that these passing planes had a "made in the USA" marking on them.[64] As the deadly bombers passed "over our heads on their way to help liberate China," Gale described her wish (and that of others) to view the planes and pilots up close.[65] In the fall of 1942, Gale noted that "with so many RAF planes and U.S. bombers in this province, we no longer fear air raids and not once all summer have we had to run to shelters." With allied assistance, Gale predicted that the Yangtze Valley might soon be returned to the Chinese and peace might be imminent.[66]

Proud that Chinese and Westerners were now actively fighting side by side in a formal alliance and determined to continue her hospital work, Gale was reluctant to leave Tzechung despite many warnings. The threat of political crisis, the inroads of Japanese troops in 1944, and the many evacuations which reduced the total missionary force of all nationalities to 850, led a committee of Chungking missionaries to decide that all women and children should be evacuated by late 1944: Gale protested.[67] When the American embassy at Chungking gave the order that all missionaries evacuate in early 1945, Gale was one of those who disobeyed orders.[68]

Gale did not believe that she should leave China in early 1945 because she felt genuinely optimistic about the Allies' role in restoring peace. She reported that her optimism was shared by the Chinese, who were very "hopeful that the Americans and British will be here soon in great force" and open up the Yangtze River.[69] In March of that year, Gale's positive outlook on China was so strong that it prompted her daughter Mary and her husband to consider returning with their two young children.[70]

Gale's optimism continued in July 1945, as she learned of Germany's May surrender, and informed supporters of recent reports that the Japanese were evacuating their civilians from Shanghai and that it appeared that Americans would be released from internment camps very soon.[71] In September 1945, Gale learned of the Japanese surrender, remaining optimistic about the future of mission work in China.[72]

Gale's eventual decision to leave Tzechung was owed both to her desire to join her husband, who was released by the Japanese, and to her growing consciousness of the tense political climate.[73] In late 1945, Gale became aware of what many had already admitted: American Commander George C. Marshall's efforts to establish a constitutional regime, which included the Chinese Communists, had failed, and China's Civil War was imminent.

By August 1946, Gale commented on what this meant to Tzechung, where conditions had deteriorated even for the rich. Thirteen of Tzechung's sugar factories had failed because the government had used Tzechung's transportation to ship rice to soldiers, thereby preventing the sugar manufacturers from shipping their wares to markets, and causing a financial disaster to hit the city full force.[74] Gale noted in September that Chiang Kai-shek's pictures were torn down from all Communist headquarters and that news from Chungking declared a 98 percent chance of civil war in China.[75]

To her longtime supporter Miss Burtis, Gale expressed disappointment with Chiang. No longer perceiving Chiang as a Christ figure, Gale instead emphasized his human frailties and the disproportionately heavy weight of his burdens. However, like many missionaries, she did not blame him for the deteriorating political situation in China.[76] Perhaps unwilling to discourage her supporters, Gale emphasized to Miss Burtis that she continued to believe in the generalissimo's sincere spirituality and she attempted to find solace in his penchant for daily prayer.[77] Gale's disappointment with conditions in Tzechung was targeted, not toward Chiang, but toward the corrupt Nationalist government.

Because of her experiences at Chadwick Memorial Hospital, Gale had come into contact with patients who had experienced the devastation caused by Nationalist leaders' foreign exchange racket. Gale was aware that the high cost of food and supplies in West China was a direct result of an inflation caused by an artificially high fixed rate of exchange. While poor Chinese and missionaries felt the adverse effects of this inflation, those who ran China's national bank profited, purchasing gold with cheap Chinese dollars and depositing the profits in American banks.[78]

Gale's disappointment with Nationalist leaders was also owed to the government's regulation, beginning in the spring of 1943, that there be no compulsory church attendance for mission school students and that Bible classes be held only after school hours.[79] Moreover, Christian work was far more difficult than it had been due to the fact that most educational inspectors were not Christian. Gale noted that the inspectors emphasized the three principles of Sun Yat-sen and told students that they did not need religion.[80]

Gale nostalgically recalled her early years in China, when it was "customary for all the students of our church schools to attend Sunday School and worship services." It had been rare for any girl to have graduated without having been a "real Christian," Gale remembered. Gale believed that those students around her responded wisely to the Nationalist government's orders by their formation of a "Christian fellowship" group within each institution: "We have one in the hospital, one in the girls' school, and a small group among the young men," most of whom were government high school students.[81]

Gale protested vehemently when the Nationalist government, fearing Communist infiltration, persecuted Christian fellowship groups. In 1944, Gale explained to the Methodist Episcopal Board that the "present government seems to be disliked by most folks" and that this government was aware of its reputation. Szechuan province was in a political "mess," Gale concluded.[82] The government's awareness of its own unpopularity had led to its accusations: anyone suspected of being in opposition to the government was accused of being a Communist. This affected Methodist work with young people. Gale complained that government orders came to arrest the Tzechuan high school boys who belonged to the Christian fellowship. The pastor and principal of the school protested and had the arrest called off, but the school was on the alert, careful of what they would do and say.[83]

Gale's correspondence with supporters did not significantly emphasize the Nationalist's anti-Christian activities, but focused instead on how Christianity thrived in unoccupied China. Gale explained that impetus for this growth had begun with the Sino-Japanese War and gained strength among West China refugees. After only three months in Tzechung, Gale observed that there appeared to be something of a "mass movement" going on. Students in the Tzechung girls' school who had previously refused to consider Christ now had "completely turned around." So many girls had asked for Bibles, and to join the church on probation, that it had "taxed the time of the faculty and the supply of bibles" had run short. Motivated to introduce Christianity to hospital patients, groups of girls joined together to sing in the hospital on Sunday mornings.[84]

By the fall of 1943, Gale reported that the Tzechung girls' school students had responded aggressively to the anti-Christian slogans of the Nationalists' educational inspectors. Gale reported that fifty girls decided to consecrate a room and hold a ceremony. Gale emphasized not so much the altar and cross used by the girls, but the "very beautiful service especially when each girl lighted her candle from the emblem of the true light of life and bore it forth to lighten others lives," which for Gale, represented social Christianity. Soon afterward, six girls were baptized and a large group was preparing for probationary membership.[85]

Gale believed that responsibility for the Christianizing of Chinese was owed to the superiority and excellence of her hospital. Gale attributed increasing numbers of girls' affinity for Christianity to the Chadwick Hospital's success at curing illness. Through Western medicine, Gale explained, the girls at the school had changed their thinking about Christianity, despite pressure from their government.[86] She noted to supporters that in the history of the hospital, there had never been such a well attended chapel because there were unprecedented numbers of patients, all of whom had never had better care.[87]

As the Sino-Japanese War drew to a close, Gale reported on the large numbers of patients who had "taken to coming to our daily chapel service." Earnestly curious, these were all "educated men of the business type." Some would borrow New Testaments, return to their hospital rooms and engage in interesting discussions afterward.[88]

For example, supporters learned of one young man who had declared himself a Communist, yet soon came under the influence of missionary education and the hospital, becoming a good samaritan. He had been one of many young men who worked in nearby banks and offices and attended an English class run by the missionaries. Later he occasionally began to attend church services, then the Sunday morning English Bible class. Shortly thereafter, his bank transferred the man to a neighboring city, where he soon became very ill with high fever. Showing his faith in Gale's hospital, the man boarded the bus for an uncomfortable two-hour ride, stating that if he were going to be sick, then there "was only one place for him and that was back in our Tzechung Christian Hospital." Gale noted that the man's espousal of Christianity went beyond ritual: he left forty thousand dollars in a package, to be used by the hospital for the care of the very poor.[89]

What did Gale hope that Christianity would do for the Chinese? In the case of the businessmen and self-proclaimed Communist-turned-

Christian, Gale evidently hoped that it would produce a number of socially conscious, active Chinese. Remarking upon the girls, eager to read the Bible and sing on Sundays, Gale hoped that they would come to know Jesus as a personal savior, one who would help them through life's difficult ordeals. She hoped that the song "What a friend we have in Jesus" would "sink deeply into some heart and bear fruit."[90] In short, Gale hoped that Christianity would empower men and women, and inspire them to social activism.

While Gale wanted Christianity to do the same for the Chinese as it had done for her, she often suggested to supporters that Christianity in China produced results superior to Christianity in America. In part this was because she believed certain aspects of Chinese culture superior to that of Americans'. She described the Chinese as more generous than Americans. Two of her "best friends," the "district Superintendent and his wife," were the most "kind and helpful . . . wise and discreet" people she knew. He was the chairman of the hospital board and Gale was always sure of his cooperation and help. Expressing respect for the Chinese customs, Gale pointed to the makeup of the man's household as testimony to his generosity. It was comprised of an adopted daughter, a third wife, a little grandson, the district superintendent's ninety-four-year-old mother and the adopted mother of the district superintendent's second wife. The seventy-one-year-old adopted mother had been an invalid, and had received "great care" in the man's home. When she died, Gale remarked that her funeral was an even greater reflection of the superiority of Chinese generosity over Western.[91]

At the mother-in-law's funeral everything was centered on the needs of the guests. A feast and breakfast were held for those who had come to pay their respects, and at the end, all were graciously invited to accompany the funeral procession to the Christian cemetery, over three miles outside the city. Gale compared this selflessness to Western funeral services, which emphasized the needs of the mourners, rather than guests.[92]

Gale offered supporters another example of Chinese generosity wedded to Christian influence in 1944, when she described the plight of a man who needed a foot operation but was without money or family. His neighbors, who had been begging so that the man might live on rice, approached the hospital to negotiate a deal: they would continue to raise money for his food if the man could have the necessary foot operation. The neighbors were so poor that it was difficult for them to feed themselves, Gale noted. Among the poor helpful neighbors was the family Gale had treated successfully for hookworm. Just as Gale had cured the family, who was now doing fine, the man would leave the hospital and presumably perform his own good deeds. Gale noted that, once healed, the man immediately "found his way to the chapel."[93]

It is difficult to separate the generosity stemming from those Chinese who had been exposed to Christianity from that which Gale attributed as natural to Chinese culture. Gale described to supporters how two married medical workers, Dr. Fritz Fisher and Emmy Fisher, a laboratory technician, were saved from death by many heroic Chinese who risked their lives to help them escape. The couple had converted from Judaism to Christianity prior to their departure from Vienna to Shanghai. They left Austria before the ban on Jewish emigration, arriving at the Nanchang General Hospital prior to the order against Jewish migration to the interior of China. When the Japanese took Nanchang, Fritz Fisher was authorized to work in a Japanese clinic. On three occasions, Chinese friends tried to help the couple and their two infant daughters escape, risking their lives. When the Fishers succeeded in slipping outside Nanchang, a large reward was offered by the Japanese for their capture. Despite the size of the reward, the Chinese were loyal: the couple continued to receive assistance from Chinese friends, eventually arriving successfully at the Methodist Hospital in Foochow.[94]

Just as Gale appreciated those qualities inherent to the Chinese, and intrinsic to their culture, she expressed respect for traditional Chinese religions. Her appreciation for non-Christian religions was evident upon her arrival to Tzechung. As early as 1942, her letter to supporters took note of a "fine lecture she had heard on Chinese Buddhism," as well as a visit to four Mohammedan mosques. In West China, where there were "many more Buddhists and Mohammedans" than in any other part of China, Gale believed it would be helpful to learn more about these peoples' principles of worship.[95]

Gale accepted traditional Chinese religions because she had been flexible in her interpretation of Christianity, a typical Liberal Protestant: as has been stated, she allowed her daughter, Mary Gao to attend a government school during her impressionable childhood years. Perhaps responding to the Gales' emphasis upon social Christianity over theology, Gale's eldest son Spencer joined the Catholic Church in the 1930s and another, Lester, pondered dating an Adventist.[96] Gale approved of Mary Gao's marriage to a young man named Sui Fang Chen, and sought to help him secure a scholarship even though she had no knowledge of his religious proclivities or affiliation.[97]

Gale's social Christianity colored her interpretation of Chinese Buddhism. Gale respected Chinese Buddhists, but wished they would emulate Protestant Christian's social orientation, rather than Christianity's doctrines and ceremonies. In 1944, Gale noted to supporters that some Buddhists in the city of Tzechung had taken up Christian customs, singing Buddhist chants to Christian hymns, organizing Sunday Schools "after our fashion," and embarking upon a program of "Buddhist evangelism." However, Gale criticized a Buddhist priest because he had asked that expensive food and possessions be burnt and offered to the gods, when his first priority should have been to address the city's poverty problem: Gale explained to supporters that one of four of the city's eighty thousand residents were without sufficient food.[98]

At its simplest level, Gale's message to supporters throughout her years in Tzechung was that the Chinese were innately caring toward one another and that this proclivity toward social consciousness and cooperation was further spurred through their contact with Christianity, and especially with her hospital. Supporters who contributed money to the Tzechung "poor fund," poor Chinese, who negotiated deals for poorer, ill friends, and Gale, all helped to sustain women's social Christianity. Gale did not allow problems stemming from Japanese invasion, the Nationalist government's financial and anti-Christian policies, inflation and lack of money, to adumbrate her optimistic self-portrayal or that of events in China.

9

Returning to Nanchang: The Final Years

METHODIST BISHOP RALPH WARD REQUESTED IN EARLY 1946 THAT Reverend Gale visit Nanchang and Kiukiang to determine the condition of these cities and the survival of Methodist institutions within them. Gale would join her husband in Nanchang in 1947.

Just two miles from the front lines, the city of Nanchang had been occupied by the Japanese and badly destroyed.[1] Reverend Gale reported that both cities were in bad shape: Kiukiang was "a wreck," but all Methodist schools and hospitals were still standing, and in Nanchang, "70 percent of the buildings went down." The Nanchang General Hospital, where Gale had begun her medical career, had suffered much damage and had almost been completely dismantled. The houses in the Methodist compound were in bad condition and occupied by the Chinese military, while the Gales' old house now belonged to the generalissimo and was walled off from the rest of the compound.[2]

With characteristic optimism, Gale reported to Miss Burtis that Nanchang offered an auspicious future for Christianity. More people were interested in the gospel than ever before.[3] By May 1946, while Gale was still in Tzechung, Rev. Gale preached to full houses, working with the support of many old friends.[4] In Nanchang, Reverend Gale found that people were still as genial as in the past, and that the staff of "splendid leaders" in Methodist schools and in the hospital were children when the Gales left the city for Tunki twenty-five years earlier.[5]

By the time Gale joined her husband in June 1947, the Nanchang General Hospital had been repaired, cleaned, and filled to capacity with competent medical workers.[6] Believing that she was not needed by the hospital where she had begun her medical career, she offered her medical services to the 680 students at the Nanchang Boys' Academy, an institution with no nurse or doctor.[7]

During the last three years of her missionary career, Gale was plagued by ill health, and she spent much time in bed. By February 1948, less than one year after her arrival in Nanchang, Gale developed an infected kidney.[8] Despite her illness, one missionary noted that, while she had been ill and "frail," she ran the boys' clinic and saw about 200 boys each morning.[9] Among the population of about 90,000 in Nanchang, many were poor and ill individuals who had not had the good health or money to flee to West China during Japanese occupation.[10] Gale raised money for medicine for some of the poor Chinese at the boys' school.[11]

Due to her ill health, Gale spent more time than usual at her Nanchang home. Since all mission residences were looted during war, the Gales had had all their new furniture made locally.[12] Gale described her scenic surroundings: from the living and dining room windows, one could see many camphor trees, the mile-wide Kan river and the hills and mountains beyond it. In the evening the sun would set behind the hills, making a golden lane that sometimes appeared to actually touch the sailboats on the sparkling water.[13]

In the midst of Nanchang's beauty, poverty and her own physical weakness, Gale evinced a continuing enthusiasm for evangelism. In November 1948, she commented to supporters on the opinion of visiting evangelist Dr. Sherwood Eddy: of all the cities he'd seen in China, the greatest opportunity for Christianity was in Nanchang. As Nationalists and Communists began their famous two-month Huai-Hai battle, Gale asked supporters to pray that Communism would not close avenues for presenting the gospel to Nanchang residents.[14]

Aware that with Communist victory, Gale might be forced to leave Nanchang she initially sought to deny the possibility of Communist victory.[15] The battle was fought about one hundred miles north of Nanking, where Chiang directed Nationalists' tactical movements. Gale reasoned that unless there was actual fighting at Nanking, her work would go on as usual. Unaware that the Communists controlled the villages, Gale cited reports indicating that the Communists were retreating and the fighting was far away from the Yangtze.[16] By late December, however, the surviving 130,000 Nationalist forces were squeezed into six square miles and surrounded by 300,000 People's Liberation Army troops. Faced with the reality that Communist victory was imminent, Gale resolved that she had "no intention of leaving" even if the Communists came. In fact, Gale expressed the wish that Chinese reports and newspapers would stop printing inaccuracies regarding the departure of missionaries:

> Never have the missionaries in this part of China been told to leave. The American Ambassador does not think it is at all necessary for any but those with children and the sick to leave. Many who went to Shanghai are going back to their work.[17]

By 10 January 1949, the Nationalists surrendered, and three months later, on 26 April 1949, the provincial government had gone to Kan-shien, leaving the city government at their posts. Gale explained to her daughter that all questions regarding the fate of missionary work under the Communists would soon be answered, and on 21 May 1949, critical events began to unravel: as millions of dollars worth of ammunition was exploded, the large Nationalist army left the city, replaced by the smaller Red Army.[18]

Two months of anxiety and uncertainty had preceded this peaceful transfer of power. On 21 May, the Gales watched Nationalist soldiers march slowly out of Nanchang, crossing the bridge onto the road out of the city, as fireworks exploded. Because there had been a very large underground Communist group in the city for six months prior to the turn over, the change had been quiet and slow.[19]

When the Communists were firmly entrenched, the excitement began. The city was covered with posters declaring "liberation," and all students, including those in Methodist schools, went wild with joy, making their way to city headquarters for "propaganda" work and training. For hours and days at a time Communists held meetings. Students were taught Communist dances and songs, some to evangelistic tunes. Some students went further south with troops, carrying heavy loads without food for days and walking many miles.[20]

Despite the excitement and joy, Kiangsi province had seen the arrival of a million soldiers at a time when people had much less food than was adequate for themselves. Since the start of 1949 there had been an especially intense strain upon rice and vegetable supplies, compounded by a flooding so severe that all the rice along the rivers and lowlands had been inundated for months. When the Communists arrived, the summer crop was gone and the fall crop had not yet been planted.[21]

Gale told supporters of the protests of angry farmers, forced to eat leaves and grass from the hills while giving up their rice to soldiers. Gale lamented that these starving people had been anticipating their "liberation" at a time when they could say anything they wished against their government, but now that that liberation had come, they dared not "speak their minds even in whispers."[22]

Certain that her Christian social activism was the answer to all societal ills, Gale objected to Communism's most basic tenets. Gale believed that everyone should work for reasonable pay, but that some needy people deserved special treatment, therefore, she abhorred the Communist rule that everyone must work to eat. She complained: "Just how a woman with five or six small children can earn her living and support an aged father hasn't been explained yet."[23]

Like all missionaries, Gale protested Communism's irreligiosity. Gale noted to family and supporters that despite the Communist government's assurances that there was religious freedom, groups of Communists moved into the administration building of the Nanchang Boys' School, preventing Sunday School from meeting. Communist meetings with compulsory attendance were routinely scheduled on Sundays at church time. Gale's medical duties suffered as the music department of the propaganda school settled into the administration building of the Nanchang Boys' School playing drums, horns, tom-toms, and cymbals while Gale attempted to use her stethoscope. The Nanchang General Hospital underwent severe strains, as supplies from the American Red Cross and the International Relief Committee and other organizations were cut off. From the behavior of the Communists and their soldiers, Gale remarked that one would think America was at war with China.[24]

By August 1949, Gale received formal orders from the Methodist Episcopal Board that all foreign personnel be completely cut. While the Communists' policy was to refuse to issue passes to travel, officials showed sympathy for Gale's ill health, allowing her to leave. Gale's permit was granted by 7 August 1950, and on 14 August 1950 she took an airplane to New York while her husband traveled by boat with the couple's belongings.[25]

On that flight out of China, one wonders what thoughts passed through Gale's mind as she likely assessed her decades in China. Fortunately, Gale's correspondence sheds some light on this question. During the 1940s, as Gale added new supporters to her address list, and her correspondence became especially abundant, she began expressing ideas about the effects of her self-representation and her descriptions of China. Gale found it noteworthy that one supporter, on her way to address a woman's missionary group, was stopped by her postman and handed one of Gale's letters. She then took it with her and used it very "dramatically."[26]

Indeed, Gale noted that she had a larger effect than she initially realized because supporters' letters had

> started my thinking along new channels. I had not thought that we were the actors in one of life's great dramas but I suppose in the years to come some poet will be setting these scenes that we have been living into some dream for the world to see and read.[27]

Perhaps because of these realizations, beginning during the 1940s, Gale's correspondence made reference to her own image. She noted the patients' amusement at "an old lady with snow white hair and with many wrinkles, appearing here and disappearing there." She reported the observations of one group of students who said: "You never see an old Chinese lady fling around like that." Gale agreed that this was true, for after age "fifty or thereabouts you are, supposed to be a lady of leisure to be cared for by the rest of the family." Revealing her wish to change Chinese perceptions of women, and doubtlessly reacting to American prejudices against active career women, she noted that it was "great fun to get some of these young folks to thinking that maybe their mothers" should have "an active part in life."[28]

Repeating these comments in the fall of 1945, Gale noted the surprise of many Chinese, that she had made the difficult trip to the sacred temples in Mount Omei. The Chinese would all smile, she noted, "especially when we were in a village and I could walk as fast as any of them." Gale went on to postulate that Chinese women of Gale's age would have thought neither of going on a trip like that, nor of being hospital superintendent. Thus, Gale made supporters aware that she perceived herself as a role model to Chinese women.[29]

In 1946 Gale expressed happy astonishment when one "old lady," a patient whom she believed to be despondent and uninvolved, had been watching her. The woman eventually observed: "Your hair is very white and you look very old, but the way you go up and down the stairs is a wonder."[30] Indeed, several of the older ladies expressed amazement at how Gale made her way from the clinic room to the drug room to the fourth floor, engaging in a variety of duties, including overseeing repairs.[31] On one occasion, Gale observed the presence of many older women who had made a pilgrimage to Buddhist shrines in Tzechung after being told that they were too old to make the trip to the famous Buddhist temple in Shanghai. As the women came and went with their walking sticks and canes, Gale became aware of their stares, predicting that they would soon be telling stories of the "foreign woman with the snow white hair, who went racing down the street, not at all as a dignified lady of my age should do!"[32]

Of equal, if not greater joy, was Gale's self-perception as a role model for Americans. She told supporters the comment of an acting dean of St. John's Medical School when he learned of Gale's position in Tzechung and, making reference to her age, remarked: "I am glad to know that you are still able to superintend a hospital of sixty-five beds." Gale noted that she "had to laugh. . . . I shall have to reply that I am glad that he can still be the dean of a medical college despite the fact that he had retired several years ago." Clearly, Gale believed that a woman of any age had the same right as any man to be the supervisor of a hospital.[33]

Important evidence of Gale's perception of the male-female equality was evinced in her letter to her daughter Mary on the eve of her wedding.

I think marriage—true marriage is one of the most beautiful gifts of God to us. Who but God could have conceived of such a lovely institution as a Christian home where husband and wife love each other . . . and where both love God and try to serve Him . . . as well as their fellow men.[34]

Gale's attitude toward marriage was revealed more in actions than words. While Gale had always been the dutiful wife, her career had often taken a higher priority than her spousal obligations.

When Gale had the opportunity to join her husband in Nanchang after the close of World War II, she proved that her hospital duties came before her allegiance to him. The Chadwick Memorial Hospital had had no surgeon for nine months and it appeared that no Chinese or foreign doctor could be found to take over its administration. As Gale explained: "not many doctors would be willing to leave the big city for a small place like this."[35] Consequently, Gale resolved that the "Master needs me here" and she would wait until a suitable replacement was found.[36]

In trying to find a replacement, Gale's ordeal reflected her unwillingness to sacrifice finding the right candidate, preferably a woman, for her husband's wish to have her join him. Gale was anxious to find a physician who met her philosophical needs. Her appreciation for the Chinese led her to insist that her replacement be of generous Christian spirit and understand, not only the Chinese language, but also Chinese thinking.[37] Her appreciation did not lead her to demand that her replacement be Chinese. While Gale insisted that her first choice for administering the hospital was a Chinese doctor, Gale told her family and supporters that finding a Chinese doctor was difficult. She complained that for months she had written letters all over China but had been unsuccessful, as Gale was told that none was willing to go west.[38] In reality, Gale criticized some Chinese doctors as too money-hungry and materialistic, revealing a profound conservatism and discomfort with consumer culture.[39]

The evidence suggests, however, that Gale preferred a woman, and was willing to wait until she got one. For example, when Gale attempted to recruit two Chinese physicians, male and female, on scholarships in America, she told supporters that the lady physician was "even better at management of institutional work than" the man.[40] When these doctors proved unable to take the position, Gale's next preferred choice was also a woman, but a white one, Dr. Marian Manly.[41]

Gale believed that Manly was perfect for the position because she was born in Tzechung (the daughter of missionaries), had an intimate knowledge of the language and conservative populace, and also had experience running a medical facility, having opened the Chengtu Midwifery School during the 1920s.[42] Gale believed that the Chadwick Hospital would be a good opportunity for Manly: she noted the opening of the government's "fine midwifery school," and predicted that Manly's school now would only be temporary, while the Chadwick Hospital could be a "permanent thing" for her.[43] Only after Gale was freed by the knowledge that the hospital would stay open and that a competent administrator would continue to serve the populace, could she proceed to join her husband in Nanchang.

The search for a replacement at Chadwick Hospital was only one of several episodes demonstrating her belief in male and female equality. Gale asserted the message that her duties as a hospital administrator took priority over her duties as a wife in the non-threatening language of empowerment-through-piety, and this allowed her to bond with American women supporters such as Miss Priscilla Burtis. While she had only met Gale only twice, Burtis shared many basic assumptions with Gale. The two spent time together during the Gales' furlough: "How thankful I am that we were permitted to see each other again and to talk over our hopes, our work, our love, and the many things we have in common," Gale remembered of the meeting.[44] Indeed, it was through Miss Burtis, that the Queen Esther ladies continued to send contributions to Gale for over thirty years.[45]

Reverend Gale noted that Burtis was "of that generation of fine cultured folks of the Victorian period in American life." Yet, despite her identification with a period associated with female domesticity, Burtis never married, dedicating her life to social activism. Indeed, her support of Gale, an empowered woman, may have validated her own wish to rebel against female restrictions. As Reverend Gale correctly noted, "The ideals of her life and her generation influence our American life more than is evident on the surface."[46]

Gale's representation as a powerful older woman was evident in the tribute to her penned by one China Inland Missionary. Commemorating forty years of service in China, the author noted Gale's arrival to Nanchang in 1908:

> Foreign doctors were scarce and a woman doctor—that was something unheard of much less seen before. Yet the day came when this woman doctor had made a large place for herself in not only this city but in the hearts of this people from east to west.[47]

The tribute captured the opinions of some Chinese. Dr. Ch'i, superintendent of the Nanchang Methodist Hospital described Gale as a skilled surgeon and medical doctor who gave freely to all. He described her competence as a teacher: when the government passed a law stating that all who had studied at least five years with a foreign doctor would be allowed to sit for the government examination, many of Gale's students passed.

Ch'i described Gale not only a skilled doctor, but as brave as any man could hope to be. Gale gave medical service to the residents of the province of Anhwei, as well as the soldiers of both Northern and Southern armies, each of which gave memorial tablets as thanks. Dr. Ch'i noted that Gale could have gone home during the years of war, when the situation was deemed too dangerous for any woman; however, she stayed and helped wounded soldiers in Nanchang from 1937–39, then served as a "wise administrator, superintendent and treasurer as well as doctor." Remembering Gale's difficulty entering China after her last furlough in the United States, Ch'i noted that Gale had been the last woman to fly out of Hong Kong for West China on the last plane.[48]

Most important, the China Inland missionary's tribute to Gale noted the extent of her credibility among other medical professionals. Doctors at the Nanchang Methodist Hospital "counted it a privilege to be able to consult Gale in difficult cases. They looked to her for her skillful judgment."[49]

In essence, the China Inland missionary's tribute to Gale had emphasized what the empowerment-through-piety ideal had emphasized among Methodist women since the nineteenth century: through piety, women medical missionaries could acquire a competence and respect that was not often bestowed upon the small numbers of talented women doctors in the American medical field. The missionary's tribute should not be taken as proof that Gale was truly what she represented, but as evidence of why American women, conscious of their own culture's prejudice against successful, assertive women professionals, would have wanted to support the image of Gale in China.

Gale demonstrated an awareness of the limitations placed upon most American women, and saw herself, and some Chinese women, as role models for American women. She noted, for example, the work of a young, recently widowed female owner of a sugar refining plant who efficiently managed her business without any familial or outside assistance. Despite the fluctuating economy, she had made astute financial decisions, guarding against falling sugar prices by holding on to her produce until the market became more favorable. Gale observed that the confident and savvy businesswoman had between forty and sixty men working for her and that she was doing "something many American women would not dare to undertake."[50]

It is ironic that while many supporters may have perceived Gale as a role model for Chinese women and she too perceived herself as such for both American and Chinese women, she has been largely forgotten. *The Journal of the American Medical Association* recorded Gale's passing at the age of 79 in 1958, noting that she had been a medical missionary to China for many years; however, the work of Gale has been largely ignored in standard narratives of Methodist history and in scholarship which has explored the representations of twentieth century women.[51] While unknown by contemporary Americans, Gale is important because she was one of many women missionaries who raised money while in the field by promoting not only traditional but also challenging images of both the proper place of women and China. Gale represents the type of assertive, social-reform oriented, Christ-centered twentieth-century Methodist woman missionary that has remained unexamined by historians.

Gale's reportage on the Sino-Japanese war and Sino-American alliance encouraged women supporters' interest in the international realm, challenging notions of women's subjugation to the domestic, rather than global sphere. Despite its inherent assumption of Western superiority, Gale's correspondence did not suggest that the Chinese nation was weak and in need of protection. While using what many would consider traditional ideas, Gale suggested that values esteemed by women had a place in the global realm and that women had a right to extend their interest from the domestic to the international realm. Gale's representations enabled her to appeal to these values, link them to complementary aspects of Chinese culture, and consequently strengthen supporters' perceptions of a Sino-American friendship to an extent which allowed her to continue her medical activities in China. That these activities were so often unavailable to American women in medicine were an important reason for American women supporters' willingness to contribute to Gale's work in the China mission field.

Notes

INTRODUCTION

1. Kelman 1965, 581.
2. Iriye 1981, 22–23.
3. See the following excellent studies: Varg 1958; Rawlinson 1990; Jesperson 1996.
4. Garrett 1982, 222–23.
5. Regarding the numerical dominance of women, see the following: Bates 1978. James Reed (1983) argues that the sentimental images created by missionaries influenced United States foreign policy.
6. Hatch 1993; Finke and Stark 1989; Carwardine 1972. Methodist Episcopal Church divided into Northern and Southern branches in 1844 over the issue of slavery. In 1939 all branches of Methodism were reunited.
7. As of 1916, the Northern Methodists had the largest mission budget ($2.9 million) and the highest number of missionaries worldwide (1,428), leading eight other major missionary organizations. Reed 1983, table 1.
8. Thornberry 1974, 3.
9. Methodist Episcopal Church Board of Foreign Missions, Annual Report 1920, 576–78; The 1920 chart reflects the numbers of women in the Northern board; See also *China Christian Advocate* (hereafter *CCA*) January 1920, Missionary Directory, 8,11; and *CCA*, December 1921, 8–10.
10. For male Methodist reaction to women's numerical predominance, see Stockwell 1933.
11. Feminist historian Ann Russo (1991) noted that "feminism's desire to speak to and from the commonality and diversity of women requires that we acknowledge and understand the privileges of Western women's lives and examine how they are connected to the conditions of other women's lives." See "We Cannot Live without Our Lives": White Women, Antiracism, and Feminism," 299.
12. Weinstein 1990, 128.
13. Lian 1997, 61.
14. Cott 1987b, 4–5.
15. Ibid.
16. In 1984, Jane Hunter (1984) set the framework for depicting single and married women missionaries as conservative Victorians who attained a degree of freedom in China. Hunter cited the personal correspondence of one missionary who had commented that female oratory was "unnatural" and "strange" because it was a solitary achievement which demanded compromise with Victorian restrictions requiring female social dependency, 69, 176, 279.

181

17. Methodist women who were able to carve out greater roles and attain varying degrees of power through piety have been the subject of investigation by scholars beginning in the early 1980s. See Keller, Queen, and Thomas 1981–82; and Brereton 1991.

18. The ideal of "True Womanhood" emphasized that women's education should prepare them for a domestic role. The contrasting ideal of "Real Womanhood," identified by historian Frances Cogan, emphasized the need for practical education, enabling the female student to eventually earn a living under optimal conditions. I argue that the "cultivation-through-piety" ideal offered a third option, not yet considered by secular scholars of woman's history. See Cogan 1989.

19. Morantz-Sanchez 1985.

20. See Brumberg 1982.

21. See Fee 1987; and Morantz-Sanchez 1985, 309–11.

22. While no comprehensive work exists on women missionary doctors in China, a few studies have begun to explore the topic. Sara W. Tucker revealed that the Ch'ing empire's traditional gender separation served women medical missionaries well, as the Chinese considered medicine the most favorable aspect of the Christian missionary presence and that women were able to assume leadership roles "at a level very unlikely to have been available to them in any mixed-sex institution" at the turn-of-the-century. See Tucker 1989. As sociologist Carol Desmither (1987) has noted, medical work in China was not without hardships. Hospitals outside of large cities were almost impossible to adequately staff, and Chinese patients resisted treatment; however, in China, women could draw up plans for buildings, supervise construction and make sketches for hospitals and instruments. See especially 141–44; See also Gleeson 1996.

23. See chapter five of Robert 1996.

24. Gale's writings contrast with the scholarly view that women missionaries who challenged white male authority encouraged their women converts to take a subservient role to men. See Flemming 1989 and Chaudhuri 1992. The above works are in keeping with Jane Hunter's 1984 model. Hunter noted that one single woman missionary, Mamie Glassburner taught Bible verses with a message that "clearly implied that God willed patience and forebearance with the demands of church brothers," but because that study focused upon a large number of women missionaries within two Protestant denominations, the complexities of each woman were beyond that study's scope and chronological limits. Thirteen years later, Glassburner penned several articles in a Methodist periodical, and revealed that she believed that all this time her students had been "emancipated by the gospel of God." See Glassburner 1927, 9, 12. General Commission on Archives and History, Missionaries of the Des Moines Branch, Mamie Glassburner biography, 117–18, 128–29, call #1465–7–2:38.

25. Of all the Chinese women acquiring public roles, it was the thirty to forty female physicians and surgeons who excited the most "attention and interest" from observers, according to Croll 1989, 114–18.

26. Andrews 1997, especially 138 where Andrews notes that tuberculosis was much lower on the Nationalists' list of priorities.

27. Robert 1996, chapter five.

28. For examples of this scholarly view, see Jesperson 1996 and Hartmann 1982. Conversely, Leila J. Rupp (1994) offers a study of twentieth-century women's international endeavors. When internationalist women's groups are examined by secular scholars, religious women are not generally a focus of study.

1. WOMEN'S MISSIONARY SOCIETIES

1. See Mathews 1991.

2. Barclay 1950. The importance that Wesley accorded women in Methodism is described on 39.

3. Carolyn DeSwarte Gifford (1985) noted that the women who took part in the Ohio Women's Crusade of 1873–74 went from prayer meetings to demonstrating against saloon owners because they received "a baptism of power." W.C.T.U. women's conversions led them to the voting booth in the 1880s.

4. Both of these books examine the significance of female negotiation of public space: Ryan 1990; Rosenberg 1989.

5. See, for example, Brumberg 1982. This is an examination of how American evangelical women in the late nineteenth century defined and catalogued the differences between themselves and "heathen" women.

6. Chandra Talpade Mohanty criticizes categorizing women as a coherent group in "Under Western Eyes: Feminist Scholarship and Colonial Discourses," in Mohanty, Russo, and Torres 1991, 51–80.

7. Donald W. Dayton explores the significance of female Methodists Frances Willard, Lee Anna Starr, Phoebe Palmer and Amanda Berry Smith, and concludes that the nineteenth-century woman's the movement had its source in evangelical revivalism. See Dayton 1976a, chapter 8; 1976b.

8. Buckley 1885.

9. Reverend Robert King Brown 1889, 24; Tuckley 1886, which encourages Christian women to be independent and self-supporting but warns against the women's neglect of their special sphere.

10. See Sarah Butler 1904, 12–13.

11. For an example of female missionary criticism of the suffrage movement, see Montgomery 1910, 45–81; Some Methodist women were in favor of suffrage. See Hardesty 1990, which discusses the Women's Christian Temperance Union's support for suffrage.

12. Isham 1913, 20–22.

13. From 1817 to 1818 the Boston Female Society for Missionary Purposes was established, and, according to Nancy Cott, corresponded with 109 other societies of like nature. See Cott 1977, 135. However, more data regarding the size and extent of these societies is needed, according to historian Carolyn DeSwarte Gifford 1985.

14. Many trace these female organizational efforts to what is termed by religious historians as the Second Great Awakening. Donald Mathews (1969) calls it the "greatest organization and mobilization of women in American history." Mary Ryan (1981) traces the connection between Oneida Female Missionary Society and other female associational activities in Oneida County, New York with female conversions during the late eighteenth and early nineteenth centuries.

15. In 1819 male missionaries organized the Missionary Society of the Methodist Episcopal Church, sending their first missionary to the French settlers in Louisiana. See Lacy 1947, on the women's New York Female Missionary Society, see Elizabeth Mason North 1870.

16. Elizabeth Mason North 1870, 15–16.

17. In addition to ibid. see chapter 1 of Louise Josephine McCoy North 1926.

18. This information is cited in Elizabeth Mason North 1870; Louise Josephine McCoy North 1926; and also Wheeler 1881, 24.

19. Wheeler (1881) provides biographical information about the missionaries supported by the society in its first ten years, 25.

20. The society was blended with the parent society in 1863. In 1869 it would become an auxiliary to the Woman's Foreign Missionary Society of the Methodist Episcopal Church, ibid, 27.

21. Ibid., 33.

22. Isham 1936, 7–8. The school, eventually named, "Baltimore Female Academy," had an enrollment of eight by the end of its first year. When the school came under the auspices of the Women's Foreign Missionary Society in 1871 it would have approximately thirty girls enrolled. See Wheeler 1881, 33–34, 94–100.

23. Wheeler 1881, 30.

24. For a discussion of nineteenth-century religious women's social relatedness, see Hunter 1985, 69, 261–63, 279 (footnote 33).

25. The Northern and Southern branches of the Methodist Episcopal Church split in 1844 after fifteen years of ministerial and lay protestations regarding slavery. All branches of Methodism were reunited in 1939. Lacy 1948, 19–36.

26. Sarah Butler 1904, 29–30.

27. On blurring of gender boundaries during the Civil War, see Clinton and Silber 1992, and Faust 1997.

28. Dowdell's letter was written to Bishop James O. Andrew. It is considered "a classic in the history of Southern missions." Tatum 1960, 15–17.

29. Patricia Hill (1985) finds the Civil War and increased educational opportunities for women to be the factors influencing the organization of missionary societies, 35–38.

30. As Timothy Smith (1957) points out, women took active roles in camp meetings in New York City during the 1850s and 1860s, 83, 124.

31. This was part of what Nathan D. Hatch (1989) describes as the "religious populism," pervading the nation between 1775 and 1845. At this time, explains Hatch, the number of clergy went from 1,800 to 40,000, while the United States population went from 2.5 million to 20 million; the "passions of ordinary people" were aroused by the example of ministers who "proclaimed compelling visions of individual self-respect and collective self-confidence," 3–5, 49–56, 58–59.

32. See Earl Kent Brown 1981; Hardesty 1981; and Dodson 1981.

33. See Cott 1977, 147, 141, 156.

34. Brereton 1991 cites Sarah Hamilton, *A Narrative of the Life of Mrs. Hamilton* (Boston, 1803), 8.

35. Another example given by Hatch (1989) is that of Nancy Mulkey, (according to an 1812 autobiography) "a shouter," who would rise with zeal . . . and fire in her eyes . . . and would pour forth an exhortation lasting from five to fifteen minutes," 78–80.

36. Isham 1936, 7–8.

37. Clementina Butler 1929, 103–7; Isham 1936, 10–11.

38. *The Heathen Woman's Friend* 1870, vol. 1:13 (June): 100.

39. For one account of this oft-repeated story, see Isham 1936, 18–19. On the "pious consumption" of nineteenth century American women see Merish 1993.

40. Isham 1936, 18; Clementina Butler 1929, 110–11.

41. Ryan notes that "Gender dimorphism in and of itself was perhaps the dominant motif of these modern American spectacles." Ryan 1990, 43–57.

42. Merish 1993, 487; Merish gives the example of Peter Cartwright, a "popular Methodist preacher" who rode circuit on the Illinois frontier, criticizing a family for the paucity of consumer items in their home, 485–87.

43. Isham 1936, 19–21.

44. Ibid., 22.

45. Wheeler 1881, 64.

46. Rev. Robert King 1889, 14.

47. Clementina Butler 1929, 112; Isham 1936, 22–23.

48. Clementina Butler 1929, 112–15.

49. Isham 1936, 22–23; Clementina Butler 1929, 111–15.

50. Ryan 1990, 48–49, 86–87.

51. Clementina Butler 1929, 115–16. Frances Elizabeth Willard would not only utilize the speaking skills she developed with the WFMS: she also emulated some of their organizing practices when she later established the Women's Christian Temperance Union. See Willard 1883.

52. Sarah Butler 1895, 42–43.

53. Ibid., 46.

54. Ibid., 50.

55. Ibid., 23.

56. Sarah Butler 1904, 68–69.

57. Tatum 1960, 16, quoted from Dowdell's letter to Bishop Andrews.

58. Sarah Butler 1904, 69–70 and Sarah Butler n.d.

59. Sarah Butler n.d. Butler's introduction states that "slight glimpses of her domestic and social life are shown in her "Reminiscences," written for her dear friend and admirer, Mrs. E. C. Dowdell of Auburn, Alabama, 18.

60. Tatum 1960, 25.

61. White 1925, 86–94.

62. See MacDonell 1928, 111–12 for White's recollection of the meeting. On Bennett's ability to combine piety with social action, see Stapleton 1983.

63. Hill (1985) notes that women were educated so that they might be better wives, mothers or teachers, 40; See Welter 1966; and 1976b.

64. Cogan 1989, 241–47.

65. Louise Josephine McCoy North 1926, 168–69.

66. Ibid., 169–70.

67. Ibid., 168. In 1896 the word "heathen" was removed and the name of the publication was changed to *Woman's Missionary Friend*. See Herb 1994, viii.

68. Knowles 1873, 510. Mrs. Ellen J. Toy Knowles was Conference Secretary in the Woman's Foreign Missionary Society of the Newark Conference from 1877 to 1925 and for forty-seven years she was Recording Secretary to the New York Branch of the Woman's Foreign Missionary Society. Obituary, *Journal of the Newark Annual Conference of the Methodist Episcopal Church,* seventy-third session, Newark, New Jersey, March 26–March 31, 1930, 243.

69. Patricia Hill (1985) has conceded only that this knowledge "must have exercised their mental muscles," 108.

70. Hart 1879, 38.

71. Tatum 1960. Mrs. McGavock advised: "The Kingdom of God cometh not with observation," 23.

72. Ibid., 62–73. Beginning in 1878 "provision was made in the first auxiliary constitution . . . for monthly meetings for business and communication of intelligence, and for reading circles." The woman's society began publishing its magazine, the *Woman's Missionary Advocate* in July 1880.

73. Herb 1994, viii-ix.

74. Tatum 1960, 69–70.

75. Brumberg 1982, 349.

76. The 1884 address, entitled "Relation of Female education to home mission work," was included in Brown and Brown 1904, 89–95. Quote on 93.

77. White 1925, 41–44.

78. The women taking leadership roles within the auxiliaries, while unpaid, were able to achieve a sense of "self-respect and power" normally attributed to professional women, according to the definition of "professionalism" offered by Brumberg and Tomes 1982, 285.

79. Hill 1985, 3.

80. Beaver 1980, 101; Hill 1985, 47–49;

81. Methodist Episcopal Church Board of Foreign Missions, 1895, 1910, and 1920 annual reports.

82. Sarah Butler 1895, 138–39.

83. Ibid., 188–89.

84. In 1910 there were thirty-five regional women's organizations in the United States, including Baptists, Congregationalists, Methodists and Presbyterians. Brumberg 1982, 351.

85. Hill 1985, 48–49.

86. At the yearly meeting of each executive committee of the WFMS, the reports from each society at home and missions on the field were assessed, the funds in the treasuries of the various branches were appropriated and the new missionaries were employed and designated to their fields. Isham 1936, 21, 26–27.

87. Other women's missionary societies were merged with denominational mission boards in the 1920s, but the Methodist women's society retained its autonomy, according to Patricia Hill 1985, 51; foreign and home mission work of women was unified under one Woman's Missionary Council. Keller 1986, 269–70.

88. Beaver 1968, 108–9; in general, the female missionary force was 49 percent in 1830 and 60 percent in 1893, according to Welter 1978, 632.

89. *Arkansas Methodist* 15 June 1939, 3.

90. Methodist Episcopal Church Board of Foreign Missions, Annual Reports 1912, 1913, 1920, 1922, 1923, 1924, 1925, 1926, 1927, 1928, 1929, 1931, 1932, 1934, 1935, 1936, 1938, and 1939.

91. Ibid.

92. Mohanty, Russo, and Torres, 1991, 12.

93. Rosaldo 1980.

2. WOMEN MISSIONARY DOCTORS IN NINETEENTH-CENTURY CHINA

1. Factors such as "self-respect and power" are important to the definition of professionalism offered by Brumberg and Tomes 1982.

2. Kristin Gleeson's research on Presbyterian missionary doctors confirmed that the women's motivation was to serve. 1996.

3. Lacy 1948, 176.

4. These same restrictions had impeded American women from allowing male physicians to examine them. See Morantz-Sanchez 1985, 24–25.

5. Beaver 1980, 131–32.

6. Morantz-Sanchez 1985, 68.

7. Ibid., chapter 4. As Morantz-Sanchez notes, five regular women's medical colleges were established at this time, including the Woman's Medical College of Pennsylvania (1850), Elizabeth Blackwell's Woman's Medical College, in New York (1868), and three other schools in Chicago, Baltimore and Boston. Women also built dispensaries and hospitals, giving female graduates clinical training.

8. Ibid., 65–68.

9. Beginning in the 1850s, hundreds of women followed the lead of Elizabeth Blackwell's graduation from Geneva Medical College. Morantz-Sanchez 1985, 49.

10. Ibid., 66, 88, 196–97. Elizabeth Blackwell was like most women doctors, perceiving vast and innate differences between men and women. Mary Putnam Jacobi was an exception in her impatience with separate standards for women, and in her perception that women were as competent as men in the scientific realm of medicine. Jacobi believed that if women did have special strengths, they were not innate, but acquired.

11. Morantz-Sanchez 1985, 238.

12. Morantz, Pomerleau, and Fenichel 1982, 82; *Medical Women's Journal* 1939, 287.

13. Hill 1985, 43.

14. As Beaver (1980) explained, by the time that the women's foreign missions boards and societies came to be organized, "the Woman's College of Medicine of Philadelphia had weathered the antagonism of the medical profession and the general public was graduating women doctors," 152.

15. Selmon 1947.

16. Anne Ryder was born in 1836, graduating with honors from Wesleyan College, Wilmington, Delaware in 1851, where she taught from 1853–57. She became a missionary wife, opening a girls' school in Bareilly, India in 1865. Turner 1995, 59.

17. The Methodists were the first to send an unmarried medical missionary from Hale's society overseas. The work of Annie Ryder Gracey included: *Eminent missionary women* (1898), a collection of biographical sketches; *In Loving Memory of Isabel Hart* (1891), a sketch of the secretary of the Ladies China Missionary Society; *Twenty years of the Woman's Foreign Missionary Society* (1889), and *Medical work of the Woman's Foreign Missionary Society, Methodist Episcopal Church* (1888).

18. For an example of how physician and founder of the New York Infirmary, Elizabeth Blackwell utilized this argument, see Morantz-Sanchez 1985, 196–97,

19. Gracey 1888, prefatory, 1–3.

20. Morantz-Sanchez (1985) notes that some women pressed "persistently for equal treatment at established institutions," those who could afford it worked in Europe, and others worked at women's hospitals in New York, Boston, San Francisco, Chicago, Minneapolis, and New Orleans, and a series of dispensaries opened and run by women. See chapter 6, especially 166–83.

21. Epstein 1971, 41. Brack 1982, 219.

22. Wheeler 1881, 161–63.

23. Gracey 1888, 119–20.

24. Ibid., 118. Joan Brumberg (1982) notes that in the literature of "heathen female debasement, three general categories of reportage consistently emerge: intellectual deprivation, domestic oppression, and sexual degradation." The seclusion referred to by Gracey falls under the category of domestic oppression. See especially 356.

25. Gracey 1888, 119–24.

26. Morantz-Sanchez 1985, 173.

27. Gracey 1888, 124–29.

28. Wheeler 1881, 163. See the following in the *Chinese Recorder and Missionary* Journal: 1880, 11:389, Dr. Coombs married Rev. Stritmatter and departed for the United States with her husband and two children; 1882, 13:190, Protestant missions in Peking and neighbourhood, notes that Dr. Howard replaced Coombs.

29. Gracey 1888, 131.

30. Ibid., 131–34.

31. Ibid., 136–39.

32. During the Tientsin Massacre of 1870, twenty foreigners, mostly Frenchmen, and many Chinese Catholics were slain. Isham 1936, 178–79; Gracey 1888, 137.

33. The Taiping Rebellion was initiated by a village school teacher named Hong Xiuquan in 1850 and it was finally repressed in 1864, when the Ch'ing Dynasty benefited from the services of Zeng Guofan, Zuo Zongtang and Li Hung chang (1823–1901). Rebellions of the Nian bands were also suppressed by these men. See Hunt 1983, 83.

34. Fairbank 1976, 196–98.

35. Pethick was an American who left the United States after the Civil War and became an expert linguist. He stayed with Li until Li's death in 1901. Hunt 1983, 118–19.

36. Ibid., 119–21.

37. Brumberg 1982, 359.

38. Gracey 1888, 135–39.

39. Ibid., 140.

40. Ibid., 146–47.

41. Michael Hunt (1983) notes that Angell was sized up by Li Hung-tsao, a senior member of the foreign office, as "simple and honest." This assessment prompted Li Hung-tsao to agree to the Angell Treaty, which allowed the United States to "regulate, limit or suspend" but not "absolutely prohibit" the entry of laborers, 88, 101, 121; Gracey 1888, 147–48; See Lacy 1947, 176–77; and Wheeler 1881, 271–73.

42. Hunt 1983, 125.

43. Gracey 1888, 140–41.

44. Ibid., 141–42.

45. Ibid., 144–45. See the following articles in the *Chinese Recorder and Missionary Journal*: 1881, 12:392, Missionary news, which describes the Isabella Fisher Hospital of Tientsin, directed by Dr. Howard. On Howard's marriage, see 1884, 15:307, Missionary news. Howard marries Rev. A. King. On the progress of the hospital by 1917, see 1917, 48:579–90, The Present Status of Protestant Missions in Tientsin, with reference to Howard on 583.

46. Gracey 1888, 149, 150; A contemporary journal described Trask as "self-educated" and possessed of "that self-reliance which fitted her for her pioneer task. Arriving in Foochow she worked without other medical help developing entirely new work." See Selmon 1947, 56–57.

47. Wheeler 1881, 168–71, quote on 171.

48. Ibid.

49. Gracey 1888, 149.

50. Wheeler 1881, 172.

51. Gracey 1888, 150.

52. Ibid., 150.

53. Ibid., 150–51.

54. Ibid., 154–56.

55. Ibid., 164.

56. Ibid., 163–65; Wheeler 1881, 173; and Lacy 1947, 177.

57. Gracey 1888, 157–67.

58. Ibid., 161–62.

59. Ibid., 170.

60. Wheeler 1881, 282–84; Gracey 1888, 172–73.

61. Trask's and Sparr's treatments of Chinese patients were reported in the missionary news, segment of *The Chinese Recorder and Missionary Journal* in 1881, 12:74. At the inauguration of the Foochow Woman and Children's Hospital in 1877, Dr. Baldwin had noted that Trask's yearly average while at the dispensary on Parent Board premises had been 1,200 cases, Gracey 1888, 154, 173.

62. Ibid., 28–30.

63. Selmon 1947, 48.

64. Gracey 1888, 33. Gracey does not indicate the identity of the "high medical authority" in America.

65. Ibid.

66. Gracey 1888, 30.

67. Cogan 1989, 241–47.

68. Selmon 1947, 48; Morantz 1982, 20.

3. AILIE GALE: THE AMERICAN SETTING

1. According to Peter Filene (1974), a "revised feminism" emerged in the 1920s. A survey of 650 career women across the country revealed that three-fourths of husbands were taking a share of household chores, and the stereotype of "a man's home as his castle," was competing with the modern image of the family as a partnership. Especially 141, 163.

2. Ailie Gale was in Nanchang, Kiangsi, 1908–21, Tunki, Anhui, 1923–27, the Shanghai American School 1927–33, Nanking, 1933–39, Tzechow, Tzechung 1941–48, and Nanchang 1948–50. General Board of Global Ministries, (hereafter GBGM), biographical file, microfilm #57.

3. As 66 percent of the Methodist missionary force, women made a noteworthy contribution to the letters reaching America from China. For just a few of the many existing examples of prolific Methodist women writers, see the following GBGM microfilms: #59, Evaline Gaw file; #58, Mrs. Theron Illick file; #45, Susan Skinner, Skinner file; #54, Mrs. Saidie Hoose, Hoose file.

4. Russo 1991, 298.

5. Issues of social concern are not always exclusively feminine. For example, Mariana Valverde (1991) illustrates how many male clergy, politicians and bureaucrats sought to create a white Protestant Canada through a self-defined social purity movement which emphasized healthy sexuality instead of the sexual repression commonly associated with traditional womanhood.

6. The data used for this study confirms that Ailie Gale, rather than Frank Gale, was the family letter writer. See, for example, GBGM, A. E. Chenoweth to Dr. Gale, 16 June 1925, microfilm #57, 2 of 2, where Chenoweth states: "I note from our files that the letters we have received are generally signed by yourself, rather than Mr. Gale."

7. Mission Hills Church files, 1932, Parish Abroad For Your Church.

8. Missionary letters and pictures were reprinted in weekly church bulletins. See GBGM microfilm #50, Marguerite Lough Berkey file, letter, Berkey to Frank Cartwright,

17 September 1933; this practice was common among other denominations. See Kessler 1990, 78–96; and Rabe 1974.

9. Frank C. Gale Collection (hereafter, FCG Collection), Gale to Priscilla Burtis, 31 October 1923, 1 of 2.

10. FCG Collection, Gale comments sadly upon the death of Priscilla Burtis in her letter to her children of 24 September 1949, 1 of 2.

11. FCG Collection, Gale to friends, 1 April 1925, 3 of 3; Gale to Priscilla Burtis, 2 August 1935, 3 of 4.

12. See *San Francisco Examiner* 18 May 1919, Chinese honor Bay City woman, public recognition accorded work of Dr. Ailie S. Gale of Oakland by official; and FCG Collection, 31 August 1934, Gale to Sons, which mentions the many friends who read the *Pacific Christian Advocate*, 2.

13. See Hoyt 1996.

14. See, for example, General Commission on Archives and History (hereafter GCAH) Paul Rugg to Gale, 29 March 1929, Gale file, Call #1043–5–2:15. Replacing A. E. Chenoweth as associate secretary in Church cultivation in 1929, Rugg's mission was to encourage more churches to give their support to the Parish Abroad Plan.

15. GBGM microfilm #57, biographical data, Francis Clair Gale.

16. Ibid., A. E. Chenoweth to Gale, 16 June 1925, 2 pages.

17. Ibid.

18. Ibid., A. E. Chenoweth to Gale, 3 January 1929; Mission Hills Church, R. E. Diffendorfer, corresponding secretary, to Mrs. H. E. Rounds, San Diego, California, 25 October 1932.

19. GBGM, microfilm #57, George F. Sutherland, assistant treasurer, Methodist Episcopal Board, to Gale, 10 January 1934, 1 page.

20. FCG Collection, 7 January 1934, Gale to Burtis.

21. Ibid.

22. FCG Collection, Gale to Burtis, 2 August 1935, 2–3 of 4. Gale promised Burtis: "We shall send you our circular letters just the same and we shall write you personal letters and feel we are one in love and prayer even though we are not the missionaries of the Simpson Church."

23. GBGM, microfilm #57, Gale to Frank Cartwright, 28 May 1948, 1 of 2; from the FCG Collection see the following: Gale to friends, 25 August 1948, 2 of 2; Gale to children, 28 May 1948, 1 of 2; Gale to Mary and Sui Fang, 26 December 1948, 1 of 2 states that the North Carolina Church paid the Gales' salary.

24. GBGM, microfilm #57, Gale to A. E. Chenoweth, 20 July 1925, 1 page; letter, G. W. to Gale, 8 December 1921; in an 18 November 1925 letter to friends, Gale remarked that she was puzzled at how the gifts had come from people whom she could not believe had known about her hospital, 2 of 2; the addresses of contributors are included in Gale's reports of the Tunki Hospital for September 1924–September 1925.

25. Methodist Episcopal Church Board of Foreign Ministers 1945, especially pages 186–90.

26. See the financial statistics for foreign war relief expenditures and other types of aid to China in following American Red Cross annual reports: 1942, 139; 1943, 124, 125, 145; 1944, 203; 1945–1946, 177; 1947, 157.

27. GBGM microfilm #57, Gale to friends, 28 June 1944, 1 of 2. FCG Collection, Gale to friends, 21 January 1942, 2 of 2; and 13 February 1944, 2 of 3.

28. Mission Hills Church, R. E. Diffendorfer, corresponding secretary, to Mrs. H. E. Rounds, 25 October 1932. See Lodwick 1986. The index of persons mentioned in the

. Chinese Recorder includes Rev. Francis Clair Gale, but not his wife, person index, vol. 1, 162. For brief mention of Mrs. Gale in the periodical, see, for example: *The Chinese Recorder and Missionary Journal*, 1914, 45:130 and 1915, 46:726, which note, respectively, the arrivals and departures of Rev. and Mrs. F. C. Gale and their three children.

29. Methodist Episcopal Church Board of Foreign Missions 1920, 81.

30. See GBGM microfilm #36, West China missionary Florence Manly to Frank Cartwright, 6 December 1929.

31. See Woloch 1984, 283; see also Desmither 1987, 156–59; Peter Filene (1974) notes that "in every field and at every level, women earned less than men," 138–39.

32. Filene 1974, 138. Peter Filene calls this a "gospel of salvation." According to Jane Hunter (1984), most missionaries came from "humble backgrounds," 29.

33. FCG Collection, Gale to boys, 21 July 1925, 2 of 3; and 16 September 1934, 1 of 3; see Reverend Gale to Frank Gale, Jr., 10 October 1935, 3 of 3. Reverend Gale explained that his wife differed from him in her attitude toward money. She was not bothered by the fact that, by 1935, the couple had not been able to save any money toward their retirement.

34. FCG Collection, Ailie Spenser Gale, brief biography by Frank Gale, Jr., undated. Ailie May Spencer's name appears in a variety of forms: while at the University of Colorado and Cooper Medical College, she signed her name Aly. Her maiden name was consistently spelled Spencer, but in this biography appears as Spenser. See FCG Collection, Cooper Medical College registration, session 1902–05, Leland Stanford Medical College, Palo, Alto, California; Gale to children, 28 May 1948, 1 of 2.

35. Frank Gale interview by author, 5 December 1996.

36. Jane Hunter (1984) notes that 50 percent of women Methodists came from the rural midwest. They were the "children of westward migrants . . . and they identified strongly with their native heartland," 28, 40.

37. University of Colorado, Tutt Library, The *Tiger* and the *Collegian*, student newspapers of the Colorado College, mention in March of 1901 that Ailie Spencer's mother died in February and her father in March of that year.

38. Lane Medical Library. From 1858, the school had been the medical department of the University of the Pacific. However, in 1882, Dr. Levi Cooper Lane provided the funds necessary for the school's independence, a new college, and hospital buildings. In 1908, the "fledgling Leland" Stanford Junior University (est. 1891, 30 miles south of San Francisco), incorporated Cooper Medical College. According to the alumni directory of the Cooper Medical College, Spencer matriculated 15 August 1902 and was graduated 9 May 1905.

39. "Ailie Spenser Gale," 2 page biography, 2, FCG Collection. For the Student Volunteer movement, see C. Howard Hopkins's *John R.Mott, 1865–1955, A Biography*, (Grand Rapids: William B. Eerdmans publishing Company, 1979).

40. FCG Collection, Ailie Spenser Gale, 2 page biography.

41. Ibid. Gale to Frank Gale, 31 December 1933, 2 of 2, describes her attitude toward public speaking.

42. Ibid. Ailie Spenser Gale, 2 page biography, 2 of 2, from the Epworth League Department of Spiritual Work, 10 September 1903. FCG Collection.

43. Ibid., for the observations of her fellow student volunteers see Gale to Francis Gale 22 August 1904.

44. Ibid., Gale to Francis Gale, 2 September 1904.

45. Ibid., Forty years . . . what hath God wrought, Francis Clair Gale, Dr. Ailie

Spencer Gale, 1908–48, 3 of 3; Miss Anne Metz, China Inland Mission, to friends of the Gales.

46. GBGM Francis Gale file, microfilm #57. Otis Spencer Gale was born in 1906, Lester Sinclair in 1908.

47. FCG Collection, Gale would explain that her medical degree burned in the San Francisco fire of 1906. Gale to boys, 19 September 1936, 1 of 3; Frank Gale, January 1997 telephone interview with author.

48. Morantz-Sanchez 1985, 234.

49. The total number of graduates from 1877–1908 was 104. See Lane Medical Library, "Women Graduates Cooper Medical College."

50. Medicine was the only profession where there was an absolute decline in the numbers of women. Morantz-Sanchez 1985, 234; Cott 1987b, notes that after the first decade of the twentieth century, the proportion of women physicians and surgeons continued to slip nationally, 218.

51. As Peter Filene (1974) has noted, one-third of all medical schools had never graduated a woman and more than 90 percent of hospitals refused to admit female interns, 138.

52. Gale was one of eleven women in a class of twenty-four. *Nugget*, 1901 yearbook, University of Colorado, Tutt Library, 38; Selmon 1945, 51; on her post-graduate medical experience, see FCG Collection, Ailie Spenser Gale, 2 page biography, 2 of 2.

53. Cited in Janeway 1973, 128, 9 December 1923, *New York Times*, Women want to be hospital interns."

54. According to statistics gathered by the American Medical Association in 1921, "40 of 482 general hospitals permitted women to intern, though not all of these 40 had ever had a woman intern in fact." See ibid and Cott 1987b, 221.

4. The Notable Nanchang Woman Physician

1. Fairbank 1976, chapter 8, 196–219.

2. See Honsinger 1924; FCG Collection, Ailie Gale to supporters, 12 April 1912, 2 of 2.

3. Spence 1969, particularly, chapter 6, 168. *China Christian Advocate* (hereafter *CCA*), September 1915, Dedication Sleeper Davis Memorial Hospital, 11, states that President Yuan Shih-kai sent a special military band which "provided exquisite music," and a representative who made a congratulatory speech. The article notes that Yuan "has been especially sympathetic with the work at the hospital."

4. Cheung 1988, 2.

5. For a reference to this situation, see, for instance: GBGM, 10 September 1924, microfilm #37, West China missionary James Yard to Dr. John Edwards, 1 of 1.

6. Bell and Woodhead 1913, 453–65.

7. In 1920, missionary hospitals in China ranged in size from 20 to 150 beds. Cheung 1988, 21.

8. China Medical Board (hereafter CUB), Methodist Episcopal Hospital (North) Nanchang, Kiangsu, 1914–15, box 21, folder 402. Application, Dr. J. G. Vaughan. Born in 1878, Vaughan was a Titusville, Pennsylvania native. He attended Northwestern University and Medical School and had been a Wesley Hospital intern for 21 months; see also Nanchang General Hospital Report, 23 February 1915. Regarding Gale's Chinese physician, see GBGM microfilm #57, Dr. Vaughan to Gale, 15 March 1920.

9. Lacy 1947, 70; Isham 1936, 200; *CCA*, September 1929, 7.

10. Women's Division, Board of Global Ministries 1986, 6; Ida Kahn was Gertrude Howe's adopted daughter. See Isham 1936, 226. The University of Michigan at Ann Arbor was the first state medical school to accept women.

11. According to Elizabeth Croll (1989), Mary Stone related this account to Grace Seton Thompson: Stone raised the funds for supplies and equipment, then returned to Kiukiang to establish a woman's hospital. When all was ready, the mission group responsible for the hospital refused to allow her to head it. No explanation was given. She then moved to Shanghai to begin all over again, 111–12.

12. Isham 1936, 223–25; CMB, mission application for Ida Kahn, Methodist Episcopal Mission Hospital (North) Nanchang, Kiangsu, 1914–15, box 21, folder 202.

13. See the following letters from GCAH folder 1: Francis Gale to brethren, board of Foreign Missions, 25 January 1921, call #1043–5:2:15, 5 pages; from folder 2, Francis Gale to Dr. John R. Edwards, 26 August 1930, Call #1043–5–2:16, 2 pages; See also Methodist Episcopal Church 1908, Annual report, 173.

14. FCG Collection, Gale to friends, circ. 1919.

15. Ibid. Translation of merit board presented by Dr. Gale by chief of police. Chao Tai ying, Dr. Dung's Almond Forest. Yien Ngen yung, chief of police for Kiangsi Province, November 1918, 1 page.

16. Generally, women physicians in America were restricted to female specialties for the first half of the twentieth century. Morantz-Sanchez 1985, 61–62 and especially 234–35; see also Lorber 1984, 1–2.

17. FCG Collection, Dr. Dung's Almond Forest.

18. Croizier 1973, 3–19; See also Croizier 1968.

19. Fee 1987, 2, 19, 21.

20. Morantz-Sanchez 1985, 309–11.

21. *The San Francisco Examiner*, 18 May 1919, Chinese honor Bay City woman, public recognition accorded work of Dr. Ailie S. Gale of Oakland by official. According to Yuet-wah Cheung (1988), of the three dimensions of medical missionary strategy, hospital/dispensary work, medical education and public health, the last two were considered secondary. Most missions viewed hospital/dispensary work as the most important, 20–25.

22. Unschuld 1979, 20.

23. The Rockefeller Foundation had contributed funds to several Methodist hospitals, beginning in 1915. Their efforts eventually culminated in a commitment to support the Peking Union Medical College, a center for medical research and teaching. See Spence 1990, 384–85.

24. GCAH, Gale to Dr. Vaughan, 16 August 1920, 1 of 4, call #1043–5–2:15, folder 1.

25. Ibid., Gale to Dr. Blydenburgh, 2 November 1920, 1 of 2, call #1043–5–2:15, folder 1.

26. Ibid., Dr. J. Vaughan to Dr. Ailie S. Gale, 14 October 1920, 2 of 4, call #1043–5: 2–15.

27. Ibid., Francis Gale to the Methodist board for the 1921 budget, 25 January 1921, 5 of 5, call #1043–5-2:15, folder 1.

28. FCG Collection, Gale to friends, circ. 1919, 1 of 2. Letter, Frank Gale to author, 10 December 1996, 3 of 6.

29. GCAH, Gale to Dr. Vaughan, 16 August 1920, 2 of 4, call #1043–5–2:15.

30. Ibid., Gale to Blydenburgh, 2 November 1920, call #1043–5–2:15; Dr. Hattie Love, Chinese women in medicine, *CCA*, April 1917, 9–10. Love noted that the hospitals of women medical missionaries were understaffed, underequipped, underfunded and

facing stiff competition from Chinese, Japanese, British and German government medical institutions.

31. Vaughan wanted to build a small tuberculosis pavilion and another hospital for tuberculosis. CMB, report, 15 June 1914, Methodist Episcopal Mission Hospital (North) Nanchang, Kiangsu, 1914–15, box 21, folder 202. Vaughan expressed his admiration for recent scientific discoveries which, when backed by large amounts of capital, could advance the field of medicine. See, in *Chinese Recorder: Journal of the Christian Movement in China*, 1929, Missionary health, 60:4 244–51.

32. CMB report, Methodist Episcopal Mission Hospital, Nanchang, Kiangsu, 1914–15, box 21, folder 202, 15 June 1914; GCAH Dr. Vaughan to Gale, 14 October 1920, 3 of 4, Vaughan states that "I do not know that we could raise the funds for constructing that at present," folder 1, call #1043–5–2:15.

33. FCG Collection, 23 October 1921, Gale to Simpson Church, 6 of 6.

34. Ibid., Gale to friends in the Simpson Church, 2 March 1919, 3 of 8.

35. Ibid., see the following letters from Gale to friends, 16 October 1916, 2; 17 May 1919, 1 and 5 of 8.

36. Gale to WFMS and Queen Esther Circle of the Simpson Church, December 6, 1916, 2 of 2, FCG Collection.

37. See, for example, Dr. J. Vaughan to Gale, February 1, 1922, 1 of 1, call #1043–5–2:15, Drew University Archives.

38. Frank Gale to author, telephone interview, 4 January 1997; FCG Collection, letter, Reverend Francis Gale to parents, 12 January 1909, 1 of 2; letter, Francis Gale to Ottie, 13 January 1909, 2 of 2. Francis Gale told of his wife's skill in dentistry and her expertise as a surgeon. She would perform her feats in front of large crowds of fascinated Chinese observers. Francis Gale to brother James, 27 January 1909, 2 of 2.

39. Frank Gale was born in Nanchang in 1909. Another son, John Robert, was born and died in 1913. Letters from Frank Gale to author, 5, 10, and 25 December 1996 describe the family's life in Nanchang. GCAH, Francis Gale to parents, 12 January 1909; concerning Gale's hysterectomy, see Francis Gale to Dr. John R. Edwards, D.D., 26 August 1930, call 1043–5–2:16, folder 2, Drew University Archives. It was common for women missionaries to discuss their domestic arrangements with supporters. See GBGM microfilm #49, letter from Lucy Stillman to friends, 28 December 1931, 2: "My house is taken care of by a cook and an amah . . . the cook runs the coal stove, cleans the floors, does my household laundry. The amah does the mending, personal laundry, waits on tables, answers the door . . . the expense is not so great."

40. For an example of the pre-1911 view, see Arthur H. Smith's Chinese characteristics, cited by Rawlinson 1990. As Rawlinson notes, Smith's chapter headings read "like a catalogue of moral lesions—Chinese were intellectually turbid, had no nerves, nor sympathy, nor sincerity. Only the Gospel could rescue these hordes from utter perdition," 2.

41. See, for example, *CCA*, February 1919, 2, Comment and outlook, where Chinese inability to achieve national unity was compared to conditions in the United States six years after Yorktown.

42. FCG Collection, Gale to friends, 20 April 1912, 1 of 2.

43. Many philosophers have noted the correlation between the status of a nation's womanhood and its level of development. Training manuals instructed turn-of-the-century religious workers that "a nation can never rise to greatness when her women are not respected" and that "no race . . . has ever risen above the condition of its women." See Montgomery 1910, 77.

44. See *CCA*, May 1914, 5, 8, where Julia Bonafield's article, A quarter century's

growth, describes "graduates of the Soochow Girl's School" looking forward "not only to professions but political life as well;" *CCA*, April 1916, China's new woman, 3, 14.

45. Honsinger (1924) notes that "since the days of the revolution . . . schools for girls have been springing into being everywhere. The government is opening them . . . educated women are opening them," 116, 130.

46. See GMBM, microfilm #57, letter to Gale, December 1921, where Methodists in Oak Park and Chicago, Illinois request more information about Gale's adopted daughter Mary; FCG Collection 6 December 1916, Gale to friends at Simpson Church; Gale to Miss Burtis, 7 January 1922, discussing the support of a Chinese female student at Baldwin School, 3 of 3.

47. FCG Collection, Gale to friends, 17 April 1911, 2 of 2, Gale Diary, 6 February 1911 entry discusses pulling the teeth of a "very wealthy" Chinese woman, a "fine artist," 5–7.

48. FCG Collection, Gale to friends, Nanchang period, undated.

49. Ibid., 6 December 1916, Gale to the WFMS and Queen Esther Circle of the Simpson Church, 7 of 7; letter, Gale to Miss Burtis, 1 May 1917, 3 of 4, mentions sewing classes and the request for twenty-five embroidery hoops from Simpson Church supporters; Gale to the Emmanual Bible Class, Nanchang period, undated, 2–3 of 4.

50. When a child was truly abandoned, the missionary would place them in the home of a Chinese Christian worker or Bible woman. Hunter 1984, 192.

51. FCG Collection, Gale, The story of Mary Kao, undated, circ. 1929. Gale to Miss Burtis, 2 June 1929, 4 of 7, notes that Mary's education would be given support by the Simpson Church in 1929. Gale did not want Mary to attend college in the United States because she was to "learn to be of help to her people." For another account of a similar Nanchang adoption, see Honsinger 1924, 55.

52. Editorial, *CCA*, April 1914, 4.

53. *CCA*, March 1916, Comment and outlook. In, How to produce women evangelistic workers in the Chinese church, *CCA*, November 1915, Mary Eline Carleton complained that "while there are leaders among Chinese women in medicine . . . we have few if any such workers for the evangelistic work of the church," 6–8.

54. In addition to Carleton, see also Gertrude Howe who speculated that Ida Kahn and Mary Stone had prompted much of "the great popularity of the education of girls' on the part of all classes," and "especially in the eagerness shown by them for the medical profession." *CCA*, Retrospect, May 1917, 5.

55. FCG Collection, Gale to friends, 20 April 1912, 1 of 2.

56. Ibid., Gale Diary, 1912, 39–40.

57. Ibid.

58. GCAH, Francis Gale to Dr. Vaughan, 7 December 1922, call #1043–5–2:15, folder 1. Through Simpson Church supporters, Gale paid for post-graduate study and expenses while on furlough. Gale to Miss Burtis, 8 August 1923, 3–4 of 4.

5. CHINESE NATIONALISM AND PUBLIC HEALTH WORK IN TUNKI, ANHWEI

1. FCG Collection, Gale to Burtis, 11 May 1924, 2 of 8; Bishop Birney sent a twenty-five dollar donation to Gale's hospital on 1 February 1925, stating that he was "interested and wanted to help," On 11 October 1925, Gale wrote to Burtis concerning the hospital's incoming receipts: " . . . it has only taken $28 from regular funds—all the rest has come

from gifts from friends and local receipts," 3 of 8; Gale to friends, 1 September 1929, 2 of 2.

2. Milton Stewart was a premillenialist, whose contribution resulted in the sending out of "evangelistic bands on every district of the conference." The board worried that some of the beneficiaries of the Stewart fund were advancing the premillenialist theory of the Second Coming of Christ. Lacy 1947, 223–24.

3. The Gales' three older children had each gone off to school. Mary Gao had been enrolled at the Baldwin School since 1918, Lester Gale was in boarding school and the eldest, Otis, had become a seaman.

4. Methodist Episcopal Church Board of Foreign Missions, 1923 annual report. The Methodist Board's cuts in appropriations resulted in the Martins' furlough in the 1920s.

5. GBGM, microfilm #57, Gale to A. E. Chenoweth, 20 July 1925.

6. FCG Collection, Gale told Burtis that she hated to ask for money, however, "on account of the cut in appropriations this whole hospital proposition is on my hands. I am hopeful that when we are in full running order we shall be able to keep up with the expenses." 11 May 1924, 2 of 9.

7. GBGM, microfilm #57, Gale to A. E. Chenoweth, 20 July 1925.

8. FCG Collection, History of Tunki church, Wannan District, Central China, ca. 1925. 7 January 1923, Ailie Gale to Miss Burtis, refers to check sent to Gale.

9. Ibid., Gale to Burtis, 20 July 1924, 5 of 8.

10. Ibid., list, attached to letter, Gale to Burtis, 20 March 1925, requesting sheets, gauze, adhesive tape, absorbent cotton, patients' gowns, 11 of 12.

11. Ibid., Gale to Burtis, 20 March 1925, 7–8; the treasurer in New York would write to the treasurer in Shanghai, announcing that a gift had arrived for Gale's hospital. The secretary of the finance committee would then inform Gale, who would formally request a release of the monies. Gale to Burtis, 20 July 1924, 6–7 of 8.

12. Ibid., report of the Tunki hospital, 30 September 1923–30 September 1924; Gale to Burtis, 1 February 1925, mentions a church in Oregon and their twenty dollar donation, and Gale's surprise that they had even heard of Tunki.

13. Ibid., Gale to Burtis, 26 December 1924, 2. Gale tells Burtis that she was astonished that her request for these items had been fulfilled so soon; Gale to Burtis, 19 June 1925, states that when the operating room table arrives she will send a letter to the Simpson Church's Sunday School, 10 of 10.

14. Ibid., Receipt, Board of Foreign Missions of the Methodist Episcopal Church, from the Simpson Church, 14 August 1924. This particular box weighed 306 1/2 pounds.

15. Ibid., Gale to Burtis, 11 February 1926, 2 of 8.

16. Ibid., Gale to friends, 5 December 1925, 1 of 1.

17. Ibid., Gale to Burtis, 20 March 1925, 2–3 of 12.

18. Ibid., Gale to Burtis, 18 April 1925, 2–4 of 8.

19. Ibid., 5 of 8.

20. Ibid., Gale to Burtis, 11 May 1924, 2 of 8.

21. GBGM microfilm #57, report of the Tunki hospital 30 September 1924–30 September 1925. Gale also purchased a small organ for religious services in the hospital.

22. Ibid.

23. See Garrett 1974, especially 283–87.

24. FCG Collection, Gale to Burtis, 11 October 1925, 2–3 of 8.

25. Fairbank 1976. In accordance with what had been secret treaties between Japan, Great Britain and France, some high officials in the Chinese government had received loans in exchange for their compliance with the Japanese government, 230–31.

26. Ibid., 234.

27. Ibid., 236, 277, on the Communist Party/KMT Alliance, see 238–39.

28. Varg 1958, 182–84.

29. Ibid., 186.

30. FCG Collection, Gale to friends, 30 July 1925, 1 of 3, notes that "so many letters" have expressed these concerns.

31. Ibid., Gale to Burtis, 19 June 1925, 1–2 of 8.

32. Ibid., History of Tunki church, Wannan district, central China, Ailie S. Gale, undated, ca. 1929.

33. Ibid., Gale to Miss Butman, 15 February 1925, 1–2 of 8; this was repeated in Gale's letter to Burtis, 26 July 1925, 7 of 8.

34. Ibid., Gale to Burtis, 19 June 1925, 4 of 8.

35. Ibid., Gale to friends, 30 July 1925, 1.

36. Ibid., Gale to friends, 10 January 1926, 2 of 3.

37. Ibid., Gale to friends, 18 November 1925, 1 of 3.

38. Ibid.

39. Ibid., 2 of 3.

40. Ibid., Gale to Burtis, 30 December 1925, 6–7.

41. Ibid., Gale to friends, 18 November 1925, 2; Gale to friends, 1 March 1926, 3 of 3; and 14 March 1926, 1 of 2, which explains that the Queen Esther Circle "girls" raised the money by holding fairs, 1–2 of 4; Gale to Burtis, 17 May 1926, 1–2 of 4, states that the extra three hundred dollars would go toward medicine.

42. Ibid., Gale to Burtis, 28 March 1926, 4 of 8; receipt, Board of Missions from Mary P. Burtis, Simpson Church, three cases; letter, Gale to Burtis, 18 October 1926, indicates that Gale picked up the boxes in Shanghai, then sailed up the Chien Tang River, 1 of 4; the Queen Esther Circle would meet on the second Monday evening of each month. There was a Queen Esther booth and the main feature was a Christmas box for the Gales, with a plea that: "a new story to their hospital is greatly needed . . . who would like to make a Real Estate Investment . . . Bricks $1," undated.

43. The mobilization order for the Northern Expedition came on 1 July 1926, but preparations had begun months before. Spence 1990, 345–47.

44. FCG Collection, Gale to friends, 9 May 1926, 2 of 3.

45. At the Johns Hopkins School of Hygiene and Public Health, much research was conducted on practical control of diseases such as malaria and the identification and destruction of disease-carrying mosquitoes. Fee 1987, 103–4, 109–10.

46. Sanchez 1985, 309.

47. Sutton 1925, 826–32.

48. FCG Collection, Gale to friends, 1 February 1929, recalled that "Mr. Gale has always been my right-hand man in all the health campaign work and he still carries on," 4 of 4.

49. Ibid., Gale to friends, 9 May 1926, 1 of 3; 1 March 1926 stated that Mr. Shen's friendship with the chief of police would lead to "a marked restriction of opium smoking, gambling" and other related "vice," 3 of 3.

50. Ibid., Gale to Burtis, 21 November 1926, 4 of 8.

51. Ibid., Gale to friends, 2 January 1927, 2 of 4; Gale to Burtis, 2 January 1927, 2 of 4.

52. Ibid., Gale to Burtis, 2 January 1927, 3–4 of 4.

53. Ibid., Gale to Burtis, 2 January 1927, 2 of 4.

54. Ibid., Gale to Burtis, 13 February 1927, 4 of 12.

55. Ibid., Gale to friends, 10 March 1927, 3 of 4.

56. Ibid., Gale to Burtis, 13 February 1927, 4–5 to 12.

57. Ibid., Gale to friends, 1 July 1927.

58. Ibid., History of Tunki church, Wannan district, Central China, Ailie S. Spencer.

59. Ibid., *The S.A.S. Nooze*, March 1929, supplementary issue, Mr. Gale accepts position of principal of S.A.S. for year of 1929–1930, 7; The 1931 *Columbian*, another S.A.S. publication lists Frank Gale, Jr., or "Francis Gale," as a student and Reverend Francis Gale, Sr. as acting principal in 1931, 20.

60. Ibid., Shanghai American School *Columbian*, 1929, 18, states that Ailie S. Gale was school physician and preceptress.

61. Ibid., Elam J. Anderson, principal of the Shanghai American School, to Mr. and Mrs. Gale, 7 May 1929, 1 of 2.

62. It was during this period that Dr. Gale published an article based upon student examinations. See Health examination of students in the American School, *The China Medical Journal*, vol. 43 (April 1929): 366–78.

63. FCG Collection, Gale to friends, 1 January 1928, 1 of 4, states that when she was approached for the position she felt it was "impossible." "Of course, I should much prefer being up at Tunki in my little hospital."

64. Jean Troy letter to author, 28 January 1997; telephone interview, author to Louise Cate, 29 November 1996. Cate was at the S.A.S. from 1927–31. Gale was "forceful," Cate recalled, and "we did not feel compelled to call her Mamma Gale."

65. Frank Gale to author, 20 February 1997, 2 of 3.

66. FCG Collection, see the following letters: Gale to Burtis, 29 June 1927, 1 of 1; Gale to friends, 1 January 1928, 2 of 4 states that "Mr. Li, the nurse," is doing very careful work. There was a significant number of patients at the little dispensary at the church, and the expenses of the medical work were being met by local income, 2 of 3; Gale to friends, 1 February 1929 discusses the continuance of Tunki public health work.

67. Ibid., Gale to friends, 1 January 1928, 1–2 of 4.

68. Ibid., Gale to friends, 1 July 1927, 2 of 3.

69. For another example of the correlation between Nationalist revolution and notions of empowerment for Chinese women, see Glassburner 1927, 9, 12. Glassburner noted that the women and girls "emancipated by the Gospel of God" were the only ones that supported the Nationalist revolution. See also, Work and workers, *Chinese Recorder* 60:5 (May 1929), 338. Nationalists urged Honan women to join clubs and to work together to help their less fortunate sisters. When one woman refused, apparently due to domestic time constraints, she was told that she should have the authority to act independently.

70. FCG Collection, Gale to fellow workers, 25 April 1924, 1 of 3; and Gale to friends, 1 April 1925, 2–3.

71. Ibid., Gale to friends, 1 January 1928, 2 of 4.

72. Ibid., Gale to friends, 1 June 1929, 4 pages; Gale to Burtis, 24 November 1929, makes reference to Shen's bravery; see Shen's account of the incident to Mr. and Mrs. Gale, Tunki, 13 November 1929 and Gale's 1 February 1930 account to friends, 3 pages.

73. Ibid., History of Tunki church, Wannan district, central China, undated; Gale to friends, 1 September 1929, 2 of 2.

74. Ibid., Gale to friends, 1 February 1930, 2 of 3.

75. Ibid., Gale to Burtis, 24 November 1930, 3 of 4; Gale to Burtis, 22 January 1931, 2 of 2 states that she visited San Diego's Mission Hills Church and saw "many old friends, some from China, some old college friends and relatives;" Reverend Francis Gale to Frank Gale, 20 December 1931, 2 of 3; Gale to Burtis, 26 December 1931, 1 of 4.

76. Ibid., Reverend Francis Gale to friends, 3 January 1932, 3 of 3.

6. FEMALE PROTESTANT IDEALS, LIBERAL PROTESTANTISM AND CHINESE NATIONALIST IDEOLOGY CONVERGE IN NANKING

1. FCG Collection, Gale to Frank Gale, 4 September 1933, 3 pages.

2. Methodist Episcopal Church Board of Foreign Missions 1933 *Journal*, 200. Methodists began mission work in Nanking in 1883, and by 1933, supported the University of Nanking and several union institutions: University Hospital, Language School of Nanking University, School of Education of Nanking University, Nanking Theological Seminary, School for Missionaries' Children.

3. GCAH, Frank T. Cartwright to Gale, 27 January 1933, 1 page. Cartwright stated that the Methodist Board could not give Gale the salary she requested. He mentioned the temporary financial arrangement Gale undertook with the W.F.M.S., Rev. Francis Gale file, call #1043–5 2:16, folder 2.

4. The interdenominational college opened in September of 1915 with eleven girls, nine of whom were Methodists. Lacy 1947, 163. Each representative board of control donated $10,000 for the college plant and $1,500 annually. See Beaver 1980, 167–68; See also the following *CCA* articles: Elizabeth Goucher, January 1916, Ginling College, 5–6; and January 1921, 18.

5. Xi Lian (1997) explains Chinese Nationalists' impact upon the Liberal Protestantism in China.

6. Chiang Kai-shek gave his speech, calling for a "movement to achieve a new life" on 19 February 1934. Another important principle emphasized by Chiang was that China had fallen into its "present deplorable state" because it had lost sight of core Confucian conceptions of virtue. See Chu 1980, 41–45.

7. Crozier 1976, 11–12, 164–70.

8. Describing the Communists, Shepherd noted that "there is much that is good in their program and they certainly get rid of a lot of parasites and corrupt officials." In 1931, Shepherd complained that Nanking had "not shown the slightest appreciation of all China's great rural past, and they have almost completely ignored this growing group of Communists in South China." He remarked that the people have nothing to gain by leaning over toward Nanking." Thomson 1968, 79–80.

9. Chu 1980, 37–68.

10. Thomson (1968) also notes that while Shepherd was a Congregationalist, from the beginning, Methodists took an important role in the Kiangsi project, 70–73; see also Nanchang Methodist missionary William R. Johnson's report, produced at the request of the Rev. and Madame Chiang: A suggested plan for rural reconstruction work under Christian auspices in Kiangsi Province, in GBGM, microfilm #58, William R. Johnson file. On Chiang's Special Movement Force, see Chu 1980, 52–53. See also Rawlinson, which discusses China's nation-wide health program and George Shepherd 1937, 1041–43.

11. According to Samuel C. Chu (1980), these nineteen provinces included all of China proper, with the exception of Kwangtung and Kwangsi, plus the outlying provinces of Sikang, Tsinghai, Suiyan, and Chahar. In addition, 1,300 hsien had subassociations under the provincial associations," 48.

12. Thomson 1968, 76–77.

13. FCG Collection, Gale to boys, 22 March 1936, 2 of 2 states that "Sunday afternoon and my large guest room was occupied by Mr. Sheperd;" See also Gale to boys, 1 November 1936, 2 of 2. By 1911, Kuling was one of several missionary resorts, which included Mokanshan, Kuliang, Chikungshan, Chefoo and Peitaiho.

14. Ibid., Gale to boys, 31 August 1934, 2 of 2 states that George Shepherd was in Kuling in the summer of 1934, having gone to see the "Generalissimo" 14 February 1935, 1–2 of 2.

15. Ibid., Gale to boys, 1 November 1936, 2 of 2.

16. Ibid., Gale to Frank Gale, 25 October 1936, 1 of 2; and 15 November 1936, 1–2 of 3.

17. Ibid., Gale to boys, 16 February 1936, 1 of 3.

18. Thomson 1968, 53.

19. Ibid., 50–51.

20. GCAH, Dr. J. G. Vaughan, to Mrs. Gale, 23 March 1931, 2 pages, folder 2, call #1043–5-2:16.

21. Women's attention to the social and physical needs of rural Chinese predated mainstream Liberal Protestant efforts. See CCA: Woman's work on Kiukiang north and south districts, which described the training of women in hygiene and sanitation, May 1917, 6; Jessie Marriott's Teaching village women to read, March 1917, 14; Phonetic writing to be pushed, November 1918, cover, 4.

22. FCG Collection, Gale to Frank Gale, 4 September 1933; Gale to Friends, 5 February 1934, 1 of 1; Francis Gale to friends, 30 November 1935, 3 of 3.

23. Ibid., Gale to friends, 5 February 1934, 1 of 1.

24. Pulling a two-wheeled rickshaw through China's cities was one of a few options open to some of the millions of men living in poverty in Chinese cities. Spence 1990, 431.

25. FCG Collection, Gale to friends, 28 May 1934, 2 of 2; Gale to boys, 9 December 1934, 2 of 2.

26. Ibid., Gale to friends, 5 February 1934, 1 of 2.

27. Ibid., Gale to friends, December 1936, 2 of 2.

28. Ibid., Gale to Frank Gale, 17 September 1933, 2 of 4.

29. Ibid., Gale to sons, 16 September 1934, 1 of 2. After Gale's term at the Shanghai American School was over, all three of her sons would leave for the United States, never to return to China.

30. Ibid., Gale to boys, 9 December 1934, 2 of 2.

31. Ibid., Rev. Gale's recounting of the episode was a testimony to his belief in every woman's right to excell: he listened to his wife speak, and pondered "how measly was" his "bachaelor's degree in comparison" to his wife's medical degree. He noted proudly that she looked every inch the doctor while standing on the podium. Gale to boys, 24 June 1934, addendum by Francis Gale, Sr.

32. The school was originally founded by YWCA secretary Matilda Thurston. Boyd 1986, 68.

33. FCG Collection, pamphlet, Ginling College, Nanking, China, 1934, 6 of 7.

34. Ibid., Gale to Frank Gale, 5 January 1936, 1 of 2.

35. Ibid., Gale to Burtis, 15 September 1933, 3 of 4.

36. In this regard, Gale was not unlike Pearl Buck, who appreciated the Chinese "matter-of-fact attitude toward all natural functions of life." See Lian 1997, 118.

37. While at the Shanghai American School, Gale had conducted "self-examination" groups for the young girls in her dormitory counsel. According to one alumnus, Dr. Gale educated the girls on the intimacies of marriage. Phoebe Wentworth White, interview with author, 3 April 1997. In preparation for her book on the Shanghai American School, *Fair is the name*, White conducted a survey of Shanghai American School alumnae and received this response from 1929 graduate, Doris Cole Blitch.

38. FCG Collection, Gale to Frank Gale, 5 January 1935, 2 of 2; Louise Cate, an S.A.S. student during the late 1920s, recalled that Gale was "reserved." Telephone interview with author, 29 November 1996; Gale's relationship with Naomi Cartwright, daughter of

Frank Cartwright, secretary of the MECB, was an exception. Cartwright recalled Naomi's fondness for Gale, who had helped her through her difficult adolescent period during their years together at S.A.S. Frank Cartwright to Gale, 3 February 1938, 1 of 1.

39. Ibid., Gale to boys, 22 June 1935, 1 of 3. In 1925, Ginling College had amalgamated with the first Normal School of Physical Education, established by the YWCA in 1914. Boyd 1986, 66.

40. FCG Collection, Gale to friends, Christmas 1936, 1 of 2.

41. Ibid., 1–2 of 2.

42. Ibid., Gale to Frank Gale, 29 April 1934, 2 of 2.

43. Ibid., Gale to Frank Gale, 16 September 1934.

44. Ibid., Gale to Frank Gale, 26 October 1934, 4–5 of 5.

45. Ibid., Gale to boys, 4 November 1934, 2 of 2.

46. Ibid., Francis Gale to boys, 21 October 1934, 2 of 3. Mary rebelled when her father tried to load her suitcases for the trip from the hospital, where she was studying, to the Gales' Nanking home. Francis Gale, in turn, treated her like a child: "I'll settle with you about your impudence when we get home," he scolded.

47. Ibid., Gale to boys, 9 December 1934, 2 of 2; and Gale to Frank Jr., Christmas Day 1934, 2 of 2.

48. Ibid., Gale to Burtis, 23 January 1934.

49. Ibid., Gale to Frank Gale, 3 April 1936, 1 of 3; Gale to boys, 5 April 1936, 2 of 2; Gale to boys, 10 May 1936, 2, notes that Mary went on a two week public health trip.

50. Ibid., Nanking government regulations stipulated that all nurses take a mandatory three-month training course in public health. Gale to boys, 17 May 1936, 2 of 3.

51. Ibid., Gale to Burtis, 23 August 1936, 2–3 of 4; Gale to friends, December 1936, 2 of 2.

52. Ibid., Gale to Frank Gale, 31 January 1937, 3 of 3. 27 September 1937, Gale wrote to her sister-in-law Vannah Spencer: "Mary is an "excellent nurse and takes a keen interest in her work," 2 of 2.

53. Ibid., Gale to Frank Gale, 7–12 December 1937.

54. Ibid., Gale to boys, 7 March 1937, 1 of 2.

55. Ibid., Gale to Frank Gale, 31 October 1937, 1 of 2.

56. Ibid., Gale to Frank Gale, Easter 1938, 1 of 1.

57. See, for example, Higashi 1979.

58. FCG Collection, see, for example, Gale to Frank Gale, 30 July 1939, 3 of 3. Welthy Honsinger, former Nanchang missionary, visited Gale, who noted that Honsinger had been busy making speeches in the United States, and that she was consumed with finding out what Chinese women were doing. See also, Margaret H. Brown, Present status of women in the church in China, which makes note of the admission of Chinese women to all the professions. *The Chinese Recorder: Journal of the Christian Movement in China*, 67:10 (1936): 623–26.

59. FCG Collection, Gale to friends, 12 February 1937, 1 of 4.

7. EMPOWERED BY PIETY, VICTORIOUS IN WAR

1. University of Colorado, Tutt Library, *The Tiger*, The Colorado College newspaper, 21 March 1941, 3. For a discussion of the international (male) vs. the domestic, or national (female) cultural bifurcation see Kaplan 1994.

2. University of Colorado, Tutt Library, *The Tiger*, 1941.

3. Dower, 1986, 98.

4. Varg 1958, 252.

5. Iriye 1981, 22–23.

6. FCG Collection, Gale to Burtis, 19 June 1925, 4 of 8.

7. Barnhart 1987, 29–30; Iriye 1990, 227–37.

8. As Michael Barnhart (1987) notes, Japan's army and navy both had significant economic interests in Manchuria, but the army's was deeper. In 1927, for instance, the Japanese navy initiated a project to liquefy oil from coal with the assistance of the South Manchurian Railway Company. That year, Chang would refuse to uphold his agreement for Japanese construction of five new rail lines into northern Manchuria, 24–33, 29, 55–56.

9. See Jordan 1980.

10. Barnhart 1995, 95–96.

11. Barnhart 1987, 55–56.

12. The struggle against communism took priority over the war with Japan. The policy reflected the advice of German Von Seeckt, who had advised Chiang that unless there was "peace on the outer borders" and "several years of external peace" Chiang could not achieve successful military reorganization. See Chi 1982, 36.

13. The Nineteenth Route Army had become highly anti-Japanese during their stay in Shanghai after October 1931. Moreover, the army's preceding unit (prior to Shanghai) had been formed in 1921 during the Kuomintang/Communist United Front, and Chiang had not purged this unit of Communist sympathizers, as he had his forces. Coble 1991, 42.

14. Letter from Mrs. Curtis B. Plummer, former S.A.S. student to author, 27 April 1997.

15. In all, Japan suffered 3,091 casualties and 769 deaths, while China's 40,000 fighters saw 14,000 casualties and 4,086 deaths. The Nineteenth Route Army incurred 65 percent casualties, and the forces sent by Chiang, the Fifth Army suffered 35 percent. Chinese civilian losses may have been as high as 10,000 to 20,000. Coble 1991, 48.

16. Ibid., 44–45. Spence 1990, 392–94.

17. Varg 1958, 252.

18. Jesperson (1996) sheds light upon this view of China.

19. As Parks Coble (1991) has noted, the "fighting at Shanghai electrified public opinion in China." The army's leaders were "lionized in word and song," 42.

20. Beginning in May of 1933, Chiang rewarded key pro-Japanese Nationalists with promotions while making sure that anti-Japanese leaders fell from power. Ibid., 136–37.

21. Ibid.

22. FCG Collection, Gale to children, 31 August 1934, 1 to 2. She reported that the Chinese had mistaken the Hoover for a Japanese transport ship.

23. Ibid., Gale to boys, Christmas 1936, 2 of 4.

24. Ibid., Gale to boys, 5 March 1939, 2 of 3; and Gale to Frank Gale, 22 May 1938, 2 of 2.

25. Coble 1991, 174–75.

26. FCG Collection, Gale to Burtis, 22 November 1934, 2 of 2.

27. Ibid., Gale to boys, 30 November 1935, 1 of 4.

28. Ibid., Gale to boys, 16 June 1935, 1 of 4.

29. James Thomson defined the Manchukuo Incident as marking the onset of a "negative phase" of American diplomacy. The nonrecognition doctrine was a rhetorical response, reflecting U.S. disapproval, but no further action was deemed practical. Both Secretary of State Cordell Hull and Far Eastern Advisor Stanley Hornbeck sought to forestall Secretary of Treasury Henry Morgenthau's attempts at financial assistance for

the Chinese Nationalists. Thompson 1969, 22–23; FCG Collection, Gale to Frank Gale, 8 December 1935, 2 of 4.

30. Varg 1958, 240.

31. Coble 1991, 59.

32. FCG Collection, Gale to boys, 10 November 1935, 2 of 2; Gale to boys, 15 August 1936, 1 of 2.

33. While Feng had initially been a Methodist convert, he went on to ally himself with Russia from 1925–26, join Chiang Kai-shek in 1927, then turn against Chiang in 1929. Sheridan 1966.

34. FCG Collection, Gale to Burtis, 12 September 1926, 4 pages. It was common for missionaries to comment upon the good behavior of Communist soldiers. George F. Sutherland, assistant treasurer of the Methodist Episcopal Board of Missions wrote to Nanchang missionary Evaline Gaw stating that he had heard of Chinese welcoming Communists because their government was "more considerate and the taxes less than under the National Regime." GBGM, microfilm #59, 3 February 1932.

35. FCG Collection, Rev. Francis Gale to Frank Gale, 31 January 1937, 1 of 3, wrote of his wife's capabilities as perceived by the wife of a Chinese pastor. The pastor's wife, a patient at the "back-door clinic," was quoted as having said Gale had "a heart full of love for people, especially the poor."

36. Ibid.

37. Ibid., Gale to friends, 10 November 1934, 3 of 3; Francis Gale to friends, 10 November 1934, 2 of 2; Gale to Burtis, 10 July 1935, 1 of 8. The Gales spent six months as boarders before having a new house rebuilt by 10 July 1935. FCG Collection.

38. Ibid., Gale explained that a "very powerful group" had been "trying to put Chiang Kai-shek in as dictator without his consent" and that "another group have been trying to prevent this happening." Shepherd believed the latter group was responsible for the kidnapping. Gale to boys, 13 December 1936, 1 of 2.

39. Ibid., Gale to Frank Gale, 17 January 1937, 1 of 2.

40. Ibid., Gale to boys, 16 December 1936, 2 of 3.

41. Spence 1990, 419–20.

42. FCG Collection, Gale to friends, 12 February 1937, 1 of 4.

43. Jesperson (1996) has shown that since the early 1930s, *Time* Inc. had consistently shown support for Chiang's effort to elimate the Communists, and had glossed over Communist grievances against the generalissimo, providing readers with romanticized notions of Chiang as a charismatic leader, 30–32; FCG Collection, Gale to friends, 12 February 1937, 1 of 4.

44. Ch'i 1982, 41–42.

45. FCG Collection, Gale to Vannah, (Ailie Gale's sister-in-law) 27 September 1937, 2 of 2.

46. Ibid., Gale to Frank Gale, 12 September 1937, 1 of 2.

47. Ibid., Gale to Frank Gale, 31 October 1937, 2 of 2.

48. Ch'i 1982, 42.

49. Spence 1990, 447.

50. Ibid.

51. FCG Collection, Gale to Frank Gale, 17 October 1937, 2 of 2.

52. Ibid., Gale to Frank Gale, October 31, 1937, 1 of 2., FCG Collection.

53. Ch'i 1982, 47.

54. From January 1938 until 1940, Chiang would assign the Combat Area Party-Government Joint Commission the task of mass mobilization. The Guerrilla Training

Corps would train guerrilla organizers. Yeh Chien-ying was appointed deputy director because of his Communist expertise and there were a number of Communist instructors in the school. Two separate war zones coordinated guerrilla activities in the occupied areas, as the entire country embarked upon a more intensified guerrilla warfare effort. Ibid., 55.

55. Spence 1990, 448.

56. In anticipation of Japanese occupation, Rev. Francis Gale had gone off to Wuhu for emergency relief work and Ginling College departments were split up and relocated to three areas of China: Shanghai, Hankow and Hunan. This left Gale free to provide medical assistance to the Nanchang General Hospital, which she had helped to build over a decade earlier. FCG Collection, Gale to Burtis, 3 December 1937, 1 of 4.

57. Ibid., Gale to Frank Gale, Nanchang, 10 April 1938, 1, 3 of 3.

58. Spence 1990, 448–49.

59. FCG Collection, Gale to Frank Gale, 10 April 1938, 1 of 3.

60. Ibid., Gale to Frank Gale, 20 August 1938, 2 of 3.

61. GBGM, Evaline Gaw to Frank Cartwright, 24 June 1938, 2 of 3, Gaw file, microfilm #59.

62. Ibid., Evaline Gaw to Frank Cartwright, 8 July 1938, 1 of 1; and Evaline Gaw to Frank Cartwright, 3 October 1938, 2 of 2, Gaw file, microfilm #59.

63. FCG Collection, Gale to Frank Gale, 4 August 1938, 1 of 1; Kuling notes, and 14 August 1938, 1, 3 of 3.

64. Ibid., Gale to boys, 20 August 1938, 1–3 of 3.

65. Ibid., Gale to boys, 21 September 1938, 1 of 1.

66. Ch'i 1982, 50–51; Spence 1990, 450–51.

67. FCG Collection, Gale to Frank Gale, 8 January 1939, 4 of 4.

68. GCAH, Gale to friends, 4 July 1939, 4 pages. The letter was sent through a Presbyterian family going on furlough to the United States. She asked that it be mimeographed and circulated to the list of addresses kept by her son, Lester Gale, a doctor in Bakersfield, California, call #1043–5-2:16, folder 2.

69. Ibid., 1–2 of 4.

70. Ibid., 2 of 4.

71. FCG Collection, Gale to Vannah, 27 September 1937, 2 of 2.

72. Ibid., Gale to Frank Gale, 5 February 1938, 3 of 3; in Francis Gale's letter to children, March 6, 1938, Wuhu, 1 page, he notes: "You read about the steady drive the Japs are making in the war. Their superior mechanized units make possible their getting control of the railroads and highways. But from 10 to 15 miles from the highways every part of the country is in possession of the Chinese who, having adopted guerilla warfare are working havoc with Jap forces. The Japs can never win this war."

73. Ibid., Gale to children, 20 February 1938, 1 of 5; see also Francis Gale to Frank Gale, 17 March 1938, 1, "Japs have plastered" posters all around: "Call a Japanese doctor and your ills will vanish. No money is wanted." Francis asked that the letter be circulated.

74. Ibid., Gale to Burtis, 5 June 1939, 3–4 of 4.

75. Ibid., 4 of 4.

76. The Japanese people could never learn the truth because Japanese newspapers and radios lied and kept them uninformed. China, on the other hand, let her people learn truth by radio, according to Gale. Ibid., Gale to Frank Gale, 10 October 1937.

77. Ibid., Gale to boys, 18 September 1938, 1 of 2.

78. Ibid.

79. Ibid., Gale to Frank Gale, 31 October 1937, 2 of 2.

80. Ibid., Gale to Frank Gale, 24 June 1939, 2 of 3.

81. See Tuveson 1968.

82. As Michael Barnhart (1995) notes, while Prince Konoe Fumimaro, the new Prime Minister, declared him an illegitimate leader, the preference of all of Chiang's enemies was to collaborate with him over Tokyo, 114.

83. FCG Collection, Gale to boys, Nanking, 5 March 1939, 2 of 3; Gale described Chiang's bravery when confronted with possible death in Sian as proof of God's presence in his life in Gale to Frank Gale, 22 May 1938, 2 of 2.

84. Ibid., Gale to Burtis, 3 December 1937, 4 pages.

85. Ibid., Gale to Frank Gale, 4 August 1938, 3 of 3; Rev. Francis Gale to children, 6 January 1938, 1 page. Rev. Gale explains that Japanese authorities were not permitting any but consular staff to return to Nanking.

86. Ibid., Gale to boys, 20 August 1938, 1 of 3.

87. Ibid., Gale to Frank, 4 August 1938, 3 of 3.

88. Ibid., Gale, Kuling notes, Summer of 1938, 14 August 1938.

89. Ibid., Gale to friends, 20 October 1938, 1 page. Gale to boys, 30 October 1938, 2 of 3, indicates that sixty-three copies were made of the 20 October letter.

90. Ibid., Gale to Burtis, 3 December 1937, 4 pages; and Gale to Frank Gale, 13 November 1937, 3 of 3.

91. Ibid., Gale to Frank Gale, 13 November 1937, 2 of 3.

92. Ibid., Gale to Burtis, 3 December 1937, 4 pages. See also GBGM, Evaline Gaw to friends, 24 May 1938, 1 of 2, microfilm #59, where Gaw notes that "most of the staff left but Dr. Gale stood by."

93. FCG Collection, Gale to Frank Gale, 7 December 1937, 1 of 4.

94. Ibid., Gale to Frank Gale, 22 May 1938, 2 of 2; Gale to Mary Thomas, 18 June 1939, where she states that "God has known from the beginning that he has a plan for the world which cannot be finally overthrown. No nation has ever gone on a rampage such as the aggressor nations are now trying and got away with it." Gale had privately expressed this belief to her sons two years earlier, when she explained that "God says 'the task of vindication is mine. It is for me to see that evil finally does not pay.'" Gale to boys, 15 November 1936, 3 of 3, FCG Collection.

95. Ibid., Gale to Frank Gale, 24 June 1939, 2 of 3. Nanchang missionary Evaline Gaw noted that she had "never been so conscious of God's presence," nor "closer to our Chinese Christians" than during war time. GBGM, Evaline Gaw to Frank Cartwright, 18 February 1939, microfilm #59, 2 of 2.

96. FCG Collection, see the following letters from Gale to Mary: 15 March 1941, 1 of 2; 19 April 1941, 3 of 3; Ailie Gale to Miss Burtis, 30 May 1941, 2 of 3.

97. Jesperson (1996) argues that the effort to change China in the U.S.'s own image . . ."strengthened" the status quo instead of "promoting social change," xvii. He explains that his central character, Henry Luce was merely a "convenient lens" reflecting the point of view of missionaries and others who had the same optimism about China's future, xvi.

98. In addition to Jesperson, see Hunt 1987.

99. Jesperson (1996) states that "Paternalism, and all it implies about treating adults as children, lies at the root of the American attitude toward . . . China," xvii.

100. Boyd 1986, 150.

8. CHADWICK MEMORIAL HOSPITAL, TZECHUNG

1. Their route to that city had been San Francisco, Honolulu, the Fiji Islands and Manilla. FCG Collection, Ailie Gale to Miss Burtis, 2 November 1941, 1, 2 of 4.

2. By November of 1941, U.S. intelligence had cracked the Japanese Purple Code and the American military was aware that the Japanese would attack, however, they did not know where. Utley 1985.

3. FCG Collection, Gale to children, 24 November 1941, 1 of 2.

4. Ibid., Gale to Burtis, 8 February 1942, 1 of 2. Seven hundred and fifty-four American missionaries in occupied China were interned and later sent back to the United States, see Mission societies raise 20 millions, *Christian Century*, 28 January 1942, 125.

5. GBGM, Gale to friends, 2 February 1946, 1 of 3, Gale file, microfilm #57. Gale to friends, 15 December 1941, 2 pages, and January 21, 1942, 2 pages, where she describes being unable to find a means of departure out of Hong Kong. Here Gale also explains that the city named "Tzechow" would be renamed "Tzechung."

6. GBGM, report, Dr. and Mrs. Liljestrand, West China Annual Conference Board of Medical Work, Liljestrand file, 25 December 1944, 1 of 3, microfilm #36.

7. In the summer of 1939, Dr. Ruth Hemenway left her post at a Chungking Hospital because it was breaking up into small sections to escape Japanese bombing. Hemenway 1977, 204.

8. GBGM, Gale to Frank Cartwright, 12 August 1942, 1 of 1, Gale file, microfilm #57; The hospital was in its early stages in 1918, a joint venture between the Women's Foreign Missionary Society and the Parent Board. See Dr. Sven (Harry) Liljestrand to Dr. North, 12 January 1918, 1, 3 of 3, Liljestrand file, microfilm #36.

9. Hemenway 1977, 205, 211.

10. FCG Collection, Gale to Burtis, 8 February 1942, 2 of 2.

11. Ibid., Gale to friends, 21 January 1942, 2 pages.

12. GBGM, Gale file, microfilm #57, Gale to friends, December 1942, 2 pages; Ailie Gale to Miss Burtis, 7 March 1943, 2 of 2 states that she had never taken a course in bookkeeping.

13. GBGM, Gale file, microfilm #57, Gale to Frank Cartwright, 12 August 1942, 2 of 2. Gale also noted that if it had not been for all the nurses trapped in the hospitals seized by the Japanese, there would not have been a nursing shortage in West China.

14. FCG Collection, Gale to friends, 10 September 1942, 1 of 2. See GBGM, microfilm #57, Gale to Frank Cartwright, 12 August 1942, 1 of 2; Dr. Hu, an excellent, young Chinese surgeon is hospital superintendent but Gale feared that some government hospital would draw him away with a higher salary; GBGM, Liljestrand file, microfilm #36, Dr. Liljestrand to friends, September 1942, 1 page, notes that the government was conscripting nurses, as well as surgeons and public health doctors. As a result, the hospital faced a shortage of medical workers.

15. GBGM, Gale file, microfilm #57, Gale to Frank Cartwright, 12 August 1942, 2 of 2.

16. Ibid., Liljestrand file, microfilm #36, Howard Liljestrand to friends, September 1942, 1 page.

17. GBGM, Gale file, microfilm #57, and FCG Collection, British Methodist Relief Funds sent a gift for the Nurses Training School. Gale to friends, 20 January 1943, 1 of 3.

18. GBGM, Gale file, microfilm #57, and FCG Collection. Gale to friends, 10 September 1942, 2 of 2.

19. FCG Collection, Gale to Mary, 31 May 1942, 1 of 2.

20. In early 1930, the Committee on Episcopacy voted in favor of the election of Chinese Bishops. Lacy 1947, 88.

21. GBGM, Gale file, Microfilm #57, Gale to friends, Christmas 1942.

22. FCG Collection, Gale to friends, 1 September 1942, 1–2 of 2.

23. Ibid.

24. Ibid.

25. Ibid.

26. Ibid.

27. Ibid.

28. GBGM, Gale file, microfilm #57, Gale to friends, 25 April 1943, 2 pages.

29. FCG Collection, Gale to friends, 13 February 1944, 1 of 3.

30. GBGM, Gale file, microfilm #57, Gale to friends, 18 January 1947, 2 of 4.

31. She admitted to supporters that Reverend Gale had always been the bookkeeper in the family. FCG Collection, Gale to Friends, 25 December 1942.

32. Ibid., Gale to friends, 20 January 1943, 1 of 2.

33. Ibid., Gale to Frank Cartwright, 21 February 1943, 1 page.

34. GBGM, Gale file, microfilm #57, Gale to friends, 10 May 1944, 1 of 3.

35. Ibid.

36. FCG Collection, Gale to friends, 14 August 1944, 1 of 2.

37. Ibid.

38. The cost of these Red Cross items to China, Great Britain, Soviet Russia, France and Italy, amounted to $148,000,000 in expenditures from September of 1939 to June 1945. Dulles 1971, 373.

39. GBGM, Gale file, microfilm #57, Gale to Frank Cartwright, 12 August 1942, 2 of 2, reports that the prices of ward patients' board rose from $1.53 per day in May of 1942 to $6.58 in July.

40. FCG Collection, Gale to friends, 13 February 1944, 2 of 3; Gale's first mention of the hospital's receipt of Red Cross supplies can be found in her 21 January 1942 letter to friends, 2 of 2.

41. GBGM, Gale file, microfilm #57, Gale to friends, 13 February 1944, 1 of 4; Gale's 16 February 1944 letter to Frank Cartwright, 2 of 2 confirms that the hospital bills were all paid, with a $240.00 surplus.

42. FCG Collection, Gale to friends, 17 August 1946, 2 of 3.

43. GBGM, Gale file, microfilm #57, Gale to friends, 14 August 1944, 1 of 2.

44. Ibid., Gale to Alta Emgart, 10 May 1945, 1 page.

45. Ibid., Gale to Frank Cartwright, 16 February 1944, 2 of 2.

46. Ibid., 1–2 of 2.

47. Ibid., Gale to friends, 10 May 1944, 1 of 3.

48. Ibid., Gale to Frank Cartwright, 30 May 1946, 1 of 2.

49. Ibid., Gale to Frank Cartwright, 12 August 1942, 2 of 2.

50. FCG Collection, Gale to friends, 20 July 1945, 2–3 of 3. When a U.S. officer visits her hospital, Gale introduces him to the magistrate and mayor because she feels he needs to get to know the "old type of courteous Chinese" and see a real Chinese home.

51. GBGM, Gale file, microfilm #57, Gale to Alta M. Emgart, Board of Foreign Missions, 10 May 1945, 1 page.

52. Ibid., Gale to Frank Cartwright, 16 February 1947, 2 of 2.

53. Ibid., Gale to friends, 8 April 1942, 2 pages.

54. Ibid., Liljestrand file, microfilm #57, Dr. Harry Liljestrand to friends, September 1942, 1 page.

55. Ibid., Gale file, microfilm #57, Gale to Friends, August 14, 1944, 1 of 2 GBGM mic. #57 states, that " . . . the girls in the school did not accept me at first but gradually were won over." This statement indicates that she was unaware of being overly optimistic.

56. FCG Collection, Gale to friends, 5 October 1944, 2 of 3.

57. GBGM, Gale file, microfilm #57, Gale to friends, 10 May 1945, 2 of 2.

58. FCG Collection, Gale to friends, 25 June 1944, 1 of 2.

59. Ibid., Gale to friends, 20 July 1945, 2 of 3.

60. GBGM, Gale file, microfilm #57, Gale to friends, 18 January 1947, 3 of 4.

61. FCG Collection, Gale to friends, 10 May 1944, 1 page.

62. Ibid., 2.

63. GBGM, Gale file, microfilm #57, Gale to friends, 2 February 1946, 1 of 4.

64. Ibid., Gale to friends, 28 June 1942, 2 of 2.

65. Ibid., Gale to friends, 14 August 1944, 2 of 2.

66. Ibid., Gale to friends, 10 September 1942, 1 of 2.

67. FCG Collection, *Bulletin of the Committee on East Asia, offices of the Foreign Missions Conference of North America*, 156 Fifth Avenue, New York City, 17 April 1946; Ailie Gale to friends, 14 December 1944, 3 pages. GBGM, Gale file, microfilm #57, Gale to Dr. Vaughan, 18 March 1945, 2 pages, expresses Gale's confusion regarding why the Methodists should leave the province. Frank Cartwright to Gale, 18 March and 13 April 1945, notes that a section of Gale's previous letter, dealing with why she chose to remain in China, was being copied and sent to the State Department. "We are trying to help Washington know that there are points of view different from those expressed in Chungking."

68. FCG Collection, Gale to Spencer Gale, 29 April 1945, 2 of 3.

69. Ibid., 1 of 3.

70. FCG Collection, Gale to Mary and Sui-Fang Chen, March 2, 1945, 2 of 2; Mary Gao Chen and her husband had gone to the United States in 1939, intending to stay for two years. They never returned to China; Gale to Miss Burtis, 7 May 1946, 2 of 2.

71. Ibid., Gale to friends, 20 July 1945, 3 of 3.

72. Ibid., 1 of 3.

73. GBGM, Gale file, microfilm #57, Gale to friends, 6 November 1945, 1 of 3.

74. FCG Collection, Gale to Mary and Sui-Fang, 6 August 1946, 1 of 2.

75. Fearing the worst, Gale advised Mary and her family to remain in the United States. FCG Collection, Gale to Burtis, 26 January 1947, 1 of 2.

76. F. Olin Stockwell (1953) believed that the generalissimo was having difficulty breaking away from the corrupt people surrounding him.

77. FCG Collection, Gale to Burtis, 7 August 1946, 2 of 2. Methodist missionary Hilda Weiss (n.d.), expressed the view that Chiang was a good man, but his underlings corrupt.

78. Varg, 1958, 275–76. In a letter to her daughter, Gale complained that the government allowed American soldiers to get a more preferable rate of exchange than American missionaries. FCG Collection, Gale to Mary, 14 October, 1944, 2 of 2.

79. Gale to friends, 25 April 1943, 3 of 3. Gale observed that "the school was much distressed this term by an order that went out from local government prohibiting any compulsory religious teaching or even holding classes during the regular school hours. They feared it would do away with all Bible classes. But when the matter was presented and the girls were asked to enroll in Bible classes 60% signed up."

80. GBGM, Gale file, microfilm #57, Gale to friends, 25 October 1943, 3 of 4.

81. Ibid., Gale to friends, 3 November 1946, 2 of 3; see also, Gale to Burtis, 7 March 1943, 1 of 2, which discusses government restrictions against compulsory religious teaching.

82. Spence 1990, 477–78.

83. GBGM, Gale file, microfilm #57, Gale to Frank Cartwright, 5 November 1944, 1–2 of 2.

84. Ibid., Gale to friends, 8 April 1942, 2 of 2.

85. Ibid., Gale to friends, 25 October 1943, 3 of 4.

86. Ibid., Gale to friends, 5 October 1944, 1–2 of 3.

87. FCG Collection, Gale to friends, 27 August 1943, 2 of 3.

88. GBGM, Gale file, microfilm #57, Gale to friends, 20 July 1945, 1 of 3.

89. Ibid., Gale to friends, 3 November 1946, 2 of 3.

90. Ibid., Gale to friends, 8 April 1942, 2 of 2.

91. Ibid., Gale to friends, 6 April 1947, 2 of 3.

92. Ibid.

93. Ibid., Gale to friends, 25 June 1944, 2 of 2.

94. FCG Collection, Gale to friends, 8 September 1945, 1 of 5.

95. GBGM, Gale file, microfilm #57, Gale to friends, 21 January 1942, 1 of 2.

96. Gale to boys, 8 April 1934, 3 of 4.

97. GBGM, Gale file, microfilm #57, Gale to Frank Cartwright, 25 August 1941, 2 of 2. Gale to Mary, 15 March 1941, 1 of 2.

98. Ibid., Gale to friends, 9 April 1944, 1 of 2.

9. RETURNING TO NANCHANG: THE FINAL YEARS

1. Weiss n.d., 2.

2. FCG Collection, Gale to children, 17 March 1946, 1 of 3; Gale to Burtis, 10 August 1947, 1 page.

3. Ibid., Gale to Burtis, 7 May 1946, 2 of 2.

4. Reverend Francis Gale would temporarily act as superintendent of the Nanchang Hospital beginning in 1946. Ibid., Gale to Mary and Sui-Fang, 5 May 1946, 1 of 2.

5. Ibid., Reverend Francis Gale to friends, 20 November 1947, 2 of 2.

6. Ibid., Gale discusses her journey from West China to Nanchang in her letter to Mary and Sui-Fang, 6 July 1947, 2 pages.

7. Ibid., Reverend Francis Gale to friends, 20 November 1947, 2 of 2; Reverend Gale to Rob and Maude, family members in the United States, 26 February 1948, 1 of 2. Gale's health problems became severe when she arrived to Nanchang. Her husband remarked that she had very little energy and appeared "old."

8. Weiss n.d., 15.

9. Ibid., 22.

10. Ibid., 2.

11. FCG Collection, Gale to Sui-Fang, 13 October 1948, 2 pages.

12. Ibid., Reverend Gale to friends, 20 November 1947, 1 of 2.

13. Ibid., Ailie Gale to Miss Burtis and Mary Lott, 22 September 1947, 2 of 3.

14. Ibid., Gale to friends, 20 November 1948, 2 of 3.

15. Ibid., Gale to Mary, 23 November 1948, 2 pages.

16. Ibid., Gale to children, 9 December 1948, 1 page.

17. Ibid., Gale to Mary and Sui-Fang, 26 December 1948, 2 of 2.

18. Ibid., Gale to Mary and Sui-Fang, 26 April 1949, 1 of 3.

19. Ibid., Gale to children, 7 June 1949, 1 of 2; and Gale to friends, 12 July 1949, 1 of 2.

20. Ibid., Gale to friends, 12 July 1949, 1 of 2.

21. Ibid., 2.

22. Ibid.

23. Ibid., Gale to children, 7 June 1949, 1 of 2.

24. Ibid., Gale to Mary and Sui-Fang, 16 October 1949, 1 page; Gale to friends, 31 December 1949, 2 pages.

25. Ibid. See also, Gale to Mary and Sui-Fang, 27 July 1950, 1 page. Gale to friends, 20 November 1950, 1 page. FCG Collection.

26. GBGM, Gale file, microfilm #57, Gale to friends, 10 May 1945, 1 of 2.

27. Ibid.

28. Ibid.

29. Ibid., Gale to friends, September 1945, 2 of 5.

30. Ibid., Gale to friends, 10 April 1946, 2–3 of 3.

31. Gale reiterated: "If I can just make some of these youngsters see that their dear old folks can have some interest in life after they are fifty, I shall be so glad." Ibid., Gale to friends, 10 May 1946, 2 of 3.

32. FCG Collection, Gale to friends, 17 August 1946.

33. GBGM, Gale file, microfilm #57, Gale to friends, 3 November 1946, 1 of 3.

34. FCG Collection, Gale to Mary, 12 July 1941, 1–2 of 2.

35. GBGM, Gale file, microfilm #57, Gale to Frank Cartwright, 22 August 1946, 2 pages.

36. Ibid., Gale to friends, 10 April 1946, 2 of 3.

37. FCG Collection, Gale to Burtis, 25 February 1946, 1 of 3.

38. Ibid., Gale to Mary and Sui-Fang, 5 May 1946, 1 of 2. GBGM, Gale file, microfilm #57, Gale to friends, 3 November 1946, 1 of 3.

39. FCG Collection, Gale to Frank Cartwright, 10 July 1947, 1 of 2.

40. Ibid., Gale to Burtis, 13 June 1943, 1 page; Gale to friends, 17 August 1943, 1–2 of 3, and 27 August 1943, 1–2 of 3. GBGM, microfilm #57, Gale to Frank Cartwright, 9 May 1947, 1 of 2.

41. GBGM, Gale file, microfilm #57, Gale to Frank Cartwright, 16 February 1947, 1 of 2.

42. Ibid., Gale to friends, 6 April 1947, 1 of 3. See also China Records Project, Manly Family papers, Dr. Marian E. Manly, untitled essay, About the Chin I School of Midwifery, Chengtu, Szechuan, China, personal papers collection, box no. 131, group 8.

43. GBGM, Gale file, microfilm #57, Gale to Frank Cartwright, 16 February 1947, 1 of 2.

44. FCG Collection, Gale to Burtis, 8 February 1942, 1 page.

45. Ibid., Gale to friends, 22 August, 1946, 1 page. The Queen Esther ladies had contributed much toward Mary Gao Chen's needs.

46. Ibid., Rev. Francis Gale to Mary, 13 October 1946, 1 of 2.

47. Ibid., Miss Anne Metz, China Inland Mission, Forty years . . . what hath God wrought, Francis Clair Gale, Dr. Ailie Spencer Gale, 1908–1948, 4 pages.

48. Ibid., 2 of 4.

49. Ibid., 3 of 4.

50. Ibid., Gale to friends, 18 January 1947, 3 of 4.

51. *Journal of the American Medical Association*, vol. 167 (May-August 1958): 2224, 30 August 1958, obituary.

Bibliography

PRIMARY SOURCES

Manuscript Collections

China Medical Board (CMB). Records. Rockefeller Foundation Archives, Rockefeller Archive Center, North Tarrytown, New York. Methodist Episcopal Mission Hospital Nanchang, Kiangsu, 1914–15; Methodist Episcopal Mission Hospital-Wuhu, 1920–26.

China Records Project (CRP) Collection. Divinity School Library, Yale University, New Haven, Connecticut. Elizabeth Brewster Fisher Papers; William R. Johnson Papers; Marian Manly Papers.

Frank C. Gale (FCG) Collection. In author's possession. Ailie Gale correspondence, 1904–50; Shanghai American School, *Nooze*, 1929; Shanghai American School, *Columbian*, 1929, 1931.

General Board of Global Ministries, the United Methodist Church. Central Records, microfilm collections. New York, New York. Helen Bartin file, #37; Elizabeth Brewster file, #50; Francis Gale file, #57; Evaline Gaw file, #59; Saidie Hoose file, #54; William R. Johnson file, #58; Florence Manly file, #36; William McCurdy file, #37; Edith Semester file, #42; Susan Skinner file, #45; Lucy Stillman file, #49; Theron Illick file, #58; Hyla Watters file, #57; Ernest Weiss file, #59; Pearl Fosnot Winnans file, #61; James Yard file, #37.

General Commission on Archives and History, (GCAH) the United Methodist Church. Drew University, Madison, New Jersey. J.B. Fearn Paper; Frank C. Gale Papers; Mamie Glassburner Papers; Hyla S. Watters Papers.

Lane Medical Library. Archives and Special Collections. Stanford University Medical Center, Palo Alto, California. Cooper Medical College Alumni Directory, Ailie M. Spencer registration, grades.

Mission Hills Church. Files. San Diego, California. Parish Abroad letters, 1930s.

University of Colorado, Tutt Library, the Colorado College, Colorado Springs. The Nugget, college yearbook; *The Tiger, The Collegian*, student newspapers.

Personal Interviews/Correspondence with Author

Cate, Louise, former Shanghai American School student. Interview by author. 29 November 1996.

Gale, Frank, Jr., son of Ailie Gale. Interview by author. 4 January 1997.

Plumber, Mrs. Curtis B., former S.A.S. student. Correspondence with author. 27 April 1997.

Andrus, Hilda Weiss, former nurse, Nanchang Hospital. Interview with author. 15 November 1996.

White, Phoebe Wentworth, former Shanghai American School student. Interview with author. 3 April 1997.

Journals, Methodist Narratives and Personal Histories.

Bonafield, Julia. 1916. A quarter century's growth. *China Christian Advocate* (May) 5, 8.

Bradshaw, Annie Eloise. 966 *China log*. Published by author.

Brown, Oswald E., and Anna M. Brown. 1904. *Life and letters of Laura Askew Haygood*. Nashville, TN: Methodist Episcopal Church, South.

Brown, Rev. Robert King, D.D. 1889. *Life of Mrs. M. L. Kelley*. Nashville, TN: Methodist Episcopal Church, South.

Buckley, James Monroe. 1885. What Methodism owes to woman. In *Proceedings, sermon, essays and addresses of the Centennial Methodist Conference; held in Mt. Vernon Place Methodist Episcopal Church, Baltimore, Maryland, December 9–14, 1884, with a historical statement*, edited by Henry King Carroll. New York: Phillips & Hunt, 303–17.

Burstall, Sara Annie. 1904. *Christianity and womanhood*. London: Charles H. Kelly.

Butler, Clementina. 1929. *Mrs. William Butler, two empires and the kingdom*. New York: The Methodist Book Concern.

Butler, Mrs. Sarah Frances Stringfield. N.d. *Life, reminiscences, and journal, Mrs. Juliana Hayes*. Nashville, TN: Publishing House of the Methodist Episcopal Church, South.

———. 1895. *Mrs. D. H. M'Gavock: Life-sketch and thoughts*. Nashville, TN: Publishing House of the Methodist Episcopal Church, South.

———. 1904. *History of the Woman's Foreign Missionary Society*. Nashville, TN: Publishing House of the Methodist Episcopal Church South.

Carleton, Mary Eline. 1915. How to produce women evangelistic workers in the chinese church. *China Christian Advocate* (November) 6–8.

China Christian Advocate (CCA). 1912–35. Official organ in China of the Methodist Episcopal Church. Shanghai: Methodist Publishing House.

Chinese Recorder and Missionary Journal. 1868–1941, Presbyterian Press, Shanghai. From 1868 to 1886, the periodical went from bimonthly to monthly publication. It was known as: *The Chinese Recorder and Missionary Journal* until 1924 when the subheading Journal of the Christian Movement in China was added. In 1938 it added the subheading *A China Christian Journal* and, with its merging with *The Educational Review* in 1939 it became *The Chinese Recorder and Educational Review*.

"Dr. Anne Walter Fearn," Medical Woman's Journal (September 1939): 287.

Fearn, Anne Walter. 1939. *My days of strength: An American woman doctor's forty years in China*. New York: Harper and Brothers.

Gale, Ailie S., M.D. 1929. Health examination of students in the American School. *The China Medical Journal* (April) 43:366–78.

Glassburner, Mamie F. 1927. The revolution among the women and girls. *China Christian Advocate*. March, 9–12.

Gracey, Annie Ryder. 1888. *Medical work of the Woman's Foreign Missionary Society, Methodist Episcopal Church*. Boston: Woman's Foreign Missionary Society.

———. 1889. *Twenty years of the Woman's Foreign Missionary Society*. Boston: Heathen Woman's Friend.

———. 1891. *In loving memory of Isabel Hart*. New York: Press of Democrat & Chronicle.

———. 1898. *Eminent missionary women*. New York: Eaton & Mains.

Hart, Isabel. 1879. Uniform readings. *Heathen Woman's Friend*. 11:38.

Hemenway, Ruth V., M.D. 1977. *A memoir of revolutionary China, 1924–1941*. Amherst: University of Massachusetts Press.

Hollister, Mary Brewster. 1932. *Lady fourth daughter of China: Sharer of life*. Cambridge, MA: The Central Committee on the study of foreign Missions.

Honsinger, (Fisher), Welthy. 1924. *Beyond the Moon-Gate: Being a diary of ten years in the interior of the Middle Kingdom*. New York: Abington Press.

Isham, Mrs. George (Mary). 1913. Our organization and Task." In *Our work for the world*, compiled by Mrs. William McDowell. Boston: Woman's Foreign Missionary Society, Methodist Episcopal Church.

———. 1936. *Valorous adventures: A record of sixty and six years of the Women's Foreign Missionary Society, Methodist Episcopal*. Boston: Women's Foreign Missionary Society.

Knowles, Ellen J. One of Many. *Heathen Women's Friend* 5 (August 1873): 510.

Landstrom, Elsie, ed. 1991. *Hyla Doc, surgeon in China through war and revolution, 1924–1949*. Fort Bragg, CA.: Q.E.D. Press.

Lane, Ortha May. 1971. *Under marching orders in North China*. Tyler, TX: Story-Wright, Inc.

Lindsay, Mrs. Effie Grout. 1904. *Missionaries of the Minneapolis branch of the Woman's Foreign Missionary Society of the Methodist Episcopal Church*. Minneapolis, MN: Women's Foreign Missionary Society of the Methodist Episcopal Church.

Love, Hattie, M.D. 1917. Chinese women in medicine. *China Christian Advocate* (April) 9–10.

MacDonell, Mrs. Robert W. 1928. *Belle Harris Bennett: Her life work*. Nashville, TN: Board of Missions, Methodist Episcopal Church, South.

Marriott, Jessie. 1917. Teaching village women to read. *China Christian Advocate* (March) 14.

Methodist Episcopal Church Board of Foreign Missions. 1908–39. Annual Reports. New York: Methodist Episcopal Church Board of Missions.

———. 1920. *China's challenge and the Methodist reply*. Program of Advance of the Methodist Episcopal Church in China adopted at the Program Study and Statement Conference, Peking, 27 January–10 February 1920. Shanghai: The Methodist Publishing House in China.

———. 1933. *Journal of the annual meeting of the Board of Foreign Missions of the Methodist Episcopal Church*. New York: Methodist Episcopal Church Board of Missions.

———. 1945. *Report of the executive secretary of the Division of Foreign Missions to the sixth annual meeting.* 4–8 December. New York: Board of Missions and Church Extension of the Methodist Church.

Montgomery, Helen Barrett. 1910. *Western women in eastern lands: An outline study of fifty years of woman's work in foreign missions.* New York: Macmillan.

North, Elizabeth Mason. 1870. *Consecreted talents: Or the life of Mrs. Mary W. Mason.* New York: Carlton and Lanahan.

North, Louise Josephine McCoy. 1926. *The story of the New York Branch of the Woman's Foreign Missionary Society of the Methodist Episcopal Church.* New York: New York Branch, Woman's Foreign Missionary Society, Methodist Episcopal Church.

Rankin, Hattie Love. 1960. *I saw it happen to China, 1913–1945.* Baton Rouge, LA: Claitor's Book Store.

Selmon, Bertha L. Pioneer Women in Medicine, Early Service in Mission. *Medical Women's Journal* 54 (April 1947): 51–57.

Stockwell, F. Olin. 1933. Shall we leave it to the ladies? *China Christian Advocate* (May) 4–5.

———. 1953. *With God in Red China: The story of two years in communist prisons.* New York: Harper and Brothers.

Surdham, Janet, and Luella G. Koether. 1981. *Our China experience.* Prairie du Chien, WI: Howe Printing Co.

Sutlon, L. E. Objectives of medical mission work in China: Analysis of answers to a questionnaire. *China Medical Journal* 39, no. 9 (September 1925): 826–32.

Tatum, Noreen Dunn. 1960. *A crown of service, a story of woman's work in the Methodist Episcopal Church South, from 1878–1940.* Nashville, TN: Pantheon Press.

Tuckley, Henry. 1886. *Life's golden morning: Its promises and its perils; a series of Sabbath evening lectures to young people.* Cincinnati: Cranston & Stowe.

Weiss, Hilda. n.d. Nanchang General Hospital, 1939–1951. Unpublished report, Methodist Episcopal Church, Board of Global Ministries, China Program Office.

Wheeler, Mary Sparkes. 1881. *First decade of the Woman's Foreign Missionary Society of the Methodist Episcopal Church, with sketches of its missionaries.* New York: Phillips and Hunt.

White, Mary Culler. 1925. *The portal of Wonderland: the life story of Alice Culler Cobb.* New York: Fleming & Revell, Co.

Willard, Frances Elizabeth. 1883. *Woman and temperance; or the work and workers of the Woman's Christian Temperance Union.* Hartford, CT: Park Publishing.

Winans, Pearl Fosnot. 1934. Woman's College, West China Union University. *China Christian Advocate* (December) 9.

Secondary Sources

Books

Abram, Ruth J. 1985. *Send us a lady physician, women doctors in America, 1835–1920.* New York: W. W. Norton & Company.

Airhart, Phyllis D. 1992. *Serving the present age. Revivalism, Progressivism and the Methodist tradition in Canada.* Montreal: McGill-Queen's University Press.

American Red Cross. 1941–47. Annual Reports. American Red Cross, Hazel Braugh Records Center, Falls Church, VA.

Antler, Joyce. 1977. *The educated woman and professionalization: The struggle for a new feminine identity, 1890–1920.* Ph.D. dissertation, State University of New York at Stony Brook.

Barclay, Wade Crawford. 1950. *Early American Methodism, to reform the nation.* 3 vols. New York: The Board of Missions and Church Extension of the Methodist Church.

Barnhart, Michael A. 1987. *Japan prepares for total war: The search for economic security, 1919–1941.* Ithaca: Cornell University Press.

———. 1995. *Japan and the world since 1868.* New York: St. Martin's Press.

Beaver, R. Pierce. 1980. *American Protestant women in world mission: A history of the first feminist movement in North America.* Grand Rapids, MI: William B. Eerdmans Publishing Company.

Bell, H. T., and Woodhead, H. G. W. 1913. Public health. In *China year book, 1913.* London: George Routledge and Sons.

Boyd, Nancy. 1986. *Emissaries: The overseas work of the American YWCA 1895–1970.* New York: The Woman's Press.

Brack, Datha Clapper. 1982. Displaced—The midwife by the male physician. *A collection of feminist essays and a comprehensive bibliography,* edited by Ruth Hubbard, Sue Henifin, and Barbara Fried. Cambridge, MA: Schenkman Publishing.

Brereton, Virginia Lieson. 1991. *From sin to salvation: Stories of women's conversions, 1800s to the present.* Bloomington: Indiana University Press.

Brouwer, Ruth Compton. 1990. *New women for God: Canadian Presbyterian women and India missions, 1876–1914.* Toronto: University of Toronto Press.

Brumberg, Joan Jacobs. 1980. *Mission for life: The story of the family of Adoniram Judson.* New York: The Free Press.

Buck, Pearl. 1936. *Fighting angel: Portrait of a soul.* New York: John Day.

Carter, Paul. 1956. *The decline and revival of the social gospel: Social and political liberalism in American Protestant Churches, 1920–1940.* Ithaca: Cornell University Press.

Chaudhuri, Nupur, and Strobel, Margaret, eds. 1992. *Western women and Imperialism: Complicity and resistance.* Bloomington: Indiana University Press.

Cheung, Yuet-wah. 1988. *Missionary medicine in China: A study of two Canadian Protestant Missions in China before 1937.* Lanham, MD: University Press of America.

Chi, Hsi sheng. 1982. *Nationalist China at War. Military Defeats and Political Collapse, 1937–45.* Ann Arbor: University of Michigan Press.

Clinton, Catherine, and Silbur, Nina. 1992. *Divided houses, gender and the Civil War.* Cambridge: Oxford University Press.

Coble, Parks M. 1991. *Facing Japan, Chinese politics and Japanese Imperialism, 1931–1937.* Cambridge: Harvard University Press.

Cogan, Frances B. 1989. *All-American girl, the ideal of real womanhood in mid-nineteenth century America.* Athens: University of Georgia Press.

Cohen, Warren I. 1990. *America's response to China: A history of Sino-American relations.* New York: Columbia University Press.

Cott, Nancy F. 1977a. *The bonds of womanhood: "Woman's sphere" in New England, 1780–1835*. New Haven: Yale University Press.

———. 1977b. *The grounding of modern feminism*. New Haven: Yale University Press.

Croizier, Ralph C. 1968. *Traditional medicine in modern China: Science, nationalism and the tension of cultural change*. Cambridge: Harvard University Press.

Croll, Elizabeth. 1989. *Wise daughters from foreign lands, European women writers in China*. London: Pandora Press.

Crozier, Brian. 1976. *The man who lost China: The first full biography of Chiang Kai-shek*. New York: Charles Scribner's Sons.

Crunden, Robert M. 1982. *Ministers of reform: The Progressives' achievement in American civilization, 1889–1920*. New York: Basic Books.

Desmither, Carol Marie. 1987. From calling to career: Work and professional identity among American women missionaries to China, 1900–1950. Ph.D. dissertation, University of Oregon.

Douglas, Ann. 1977. *The feminization of American culture*. New York: Knopf.

Dower, John. 1986. *War without mercy, race and power in the Pacific War*. New York: Pantheon Books.

Drachman, Virginia. 1984. *Hospital with a heart, women doctors and the paradox of separatism at the New England Hospital, 1862–1969*. Ithaca: Cornell University Press.

Dubois, Ellen Carol, and Ruiz, Vicki L., eds. 1994. *Unequal sisters, a multicultural reader in U.S. women's history*. New York: Routledge Press.

Dulles, Foster Rhea. 1971. *The American Red Cross, a history*. Westport, CT: Greenwood Press.

Epstein, Cynthia. 1971. *Woman's place*. Berkeley: University of California Press.

Fairbank, John King, ed. 1974. *The missionary enterprise in China and America*. Cambridge: Harvard University Press.

———. 1976. *The United States and China*. 4th ed. Cambridge: Harvard University Press.

Faust, Drew Gilpin. 1997. *Mothers of invention: Women of the slaveholding South in the American Civil War*. 1st Vintage Books ed., New York: Vintage Books; University of North Carolina Press.

Fee, Elizabeth. 1987. *Disease and discovery, a history of the Johns Hopkins School of Hygiene and Public Health, 1916–1959*. Baltimore: Johns Hopkins University Press.

Filene, Peter. 1974. *Him/her self, sex roles in modern America*. New York: Harcourt Brace Jovanovich; second ed., Baltimore: The Johns Hopkins University Press, 1986.

Flemming, Leslie A., ed. 1989. *Women's work for women, missionaries and social change in Asia*. Boulder, CO: Westview Press.

Gleeson, Kristin Lee. 1996. Healers abroad: Presbyterian women physicians in the foreign mission field. Ph.D. dissertation, Temple University.

Hartman, Susan. 1982. *The home front and beyond: American women in the 1940s*. Boston: Twayne Publications.

Hatch, Nathan, O. 1989. *The democratization of American Christianity*. New Haven: Yale University Press.

Herb, Carol Marie. 1994. *The light along the way, a living history through United Methodist Women's Magazines*. A special report to the Women's Division, New York: General Board of Global Ministries: The United Methodist Church.

Hill, Patricia R. 1985. *The world their household: The american woman's foreign mission movement and cultural transformation, 1870–1920*. Ann Arbor: University of Michigan Press.

Hopkins, C. Howard. 1979. *John R. Mott, 1865–1955, a biography*. Grand Rapids, MI: William B. Eerdmans Publishing Company.

Hunt, Michael. 1983. *The making of a special relationship: The U.S. and China to 1914*. New York: Columbia University Press.

Hunter, Jane. 1984. *The gospel of gentility, American women missionaries in turn-of-the-century China*. New Haven: Yale University Press.

Hutchison, William R. 1987. *Errand to the world: American Protestant thought and foreign missions*. Chicago: University of Chicago Press.

Hyatt, Irwin T., Jr. 1976. *Our ordered lives confess: Three nineteenth-century American missionaries in East Shantung*. Cambridge: Harvard University Press.

Iriye, Akira. 1967. *Across the Pacific: An inner history of American–East Asian relations*. New York: Harcourt, Brace & World.

———. 1981. *Power and culture: The Japanese-American War, 1941–1945*. Cambridge: Harvard University Press.

———. 1990. *After Imperialism, the search for a new order in the Far East, 1921–1931*. Chicago: Imprint Publications.

Isaacs, Harold R. 1958. *Scratches on our minds: American images of China and India*. New York: John Day.

Janeway, Elizabeth, advisory ed. 1973. *Women, their changing roles, New York Times*. New York: Arno Press.

Jesperson, Christopher. 1996. *American images of China, 1931–1949*. Stanford, CA: Stanford University Press.

Kaufman, Gordon, D. 1968. *Systemic theology: An historicist perspective*. New York: Charles Scribner's Sons.

Kelley, Mary. 1979. *Woman's being, woman's place: Female identity and vocation and American history*. Boston: G. K. Hall & Co.

Keller, Rosemary, Louise L. Queens, and Hilah F. Thomas, eds. 1981–82. *Women in new worlds: Historical perspectives on the Wesleyan tradition*. 2 vols. Nashville, TN: Abingdon Press.

Lacy, Walter N. 1947. *A hundred years of China Methodism*. Nashville, TN: Abingdon-Cokesbury Press.

Lian, Xi. 1997. *The conversion of missionaries, liberalism in American Protestant missions in China, 1907–1932*. University Park: Pennsylvania State University Press.

Lodwick, Kathleen. 1986. *The Chinese recorder index: A guide to Christian missions in Asia*. 2 vols. Wilmington, DE: Scholarly Resources.

———. 1995. *Educating the women of Hainan: The career of Margaret Moninger in China, 1915–1942*. Lexington: University Press of Kentucky.

Lorber, Judith. 1984. *Women physicians, careers, status and power*. New York: Tavistock Publications.

Mathews, Glenna. 1991. *The rise of public woman, woman's power and woman's place in the United States, 1630–1970*. New York: Oxford University Press.

May, Elaine Tyler. 1988. *Homeward bound: American families in the Cold War era*. New York: Basic Books.

Mohanty, Chandra Talpade, Ann Russo, and Lourdes Torres, eds. 1991. *Third world women and the politics of feminism*, Bloomington: Indiana University Press, 1991.

Morantz, Regina Marke, Cynthia Stodola Pomerleau, and Carol Hansen Fenidel, eds. 1982. *In her own words: Oral histories of women physicians*. Westport, CT: Greenwood Press.

Morantz-Sanchez, Regina Markell. 1985. *Sympathy and science: Women physicians in American medicine*. New York. Oxford University Press.

Neils, Patricia, ed. 1990. *United States attitudes and policies toward China: The impact of American missionaries*. New York: M. E. Sharpe, Inc.

Norwood, Frederick A. 1982. *Sourcebook of American Methodism*. Nashville: Abingdon Press.

Rawlinson, John L. 1990. Rawlinson, the Recorder, and China's revolution: A topical biography of Frank Joseph Rawlinson, 1871–1937. 2 vols. Notre Dame, IN: Cross Cultural Publications.

Reed, James. 1983. *The missionary mind and American East-Asian Policy 1911–1915*. Cambridge: Harvard University Press.

Robert, Dana L. 1996. *American women in mission, a social history of their thought and practice*. Macon, GA: Mercer University Press.

Rogers, Everett M. 1969. *Modernization among peasants: The impact of communication*. New York: Holt, Rinehart and Winston.

Rosaldo, Michele Zimbalist. "The use and abuse of anthropology: reflections on feminism and cross-cultural understanding." *Signs* 5 (1980): 389–417.

Rosenberg, Emily. 1982. *Spreading the American dream: American economic and cultural expansion, 1890–1945*. New York: Hill & Wang.

Rosenberg, Rosalind. 1989. *Beyond separate spheres: Intellectual roots of modern feminism*. New Haven: Yale University Press.

Ruether, Rosemary Radford, and Rosemary Skinner Keller, eds. 1981–86. *Women and religion in America*. New York: Harper & Row.

Ryan, Mary P. 1981. *Cradle of the middle class: The family in Oneida County, New York, 1790–1865*. Cambridge, MA: Cambridge University Press.

———. 1990. *Women in public: Between banners and ballots, 1825–1880*. Baltimore: Johns Hopkins University Press.

Schaller, Michael. 1979. *The United States and China in the twentieth century*. New York: Oxford University Press.

Scott, Anne Firor. 1970. *The southern lady: From pedestal to politics, 1830–1930*. Chicago: University of Chicago Press.

———. 1984. *Making the invisible woman visible*. Urbana: University of Illinois.

Sheridan, James E. 1966. *Chinese warlord: The career of Feng Yu-hsiang*. Stanford, CA: Stanford University Press.

Shyrock, Richard Harrison. 1966. *Medicine in America, historical essays*. Baltimore: Johns Hopkins Press.

Smith, Timothy. 1957. *Revivalism and social reform: American Protestantism on the eve of the Civil War*. Nashville, TN: Abingdon Press.

Spence, Jonathan. 1969. *To change China: Western advisers in China 1620–1960*. Boston: Little, Brown.

————. 1990. *The search for modern China*. New York: W. W. Norton & Co.

Thomson, James Jr. 1968. *While China faced west, America reformers in Nationalist China, 1928–1937*. Cambridge: Harvard University Press.

Thornberry, Milo Lancaster. 1974. American missionaries and the Chinese Communists: A study of views expressed by Methodist Episcopal Church Missionaries, 1921–1941. Ph.D. dissertation. Boston University School of Theology.

Turner, Kristen D. 1995. *A guide to materials on women in the United Methodist Church archives*. Madison, New Jersey: General Commission on Archives and History. The United Methodist Episcopal Church.

Tuveson, Ernest Lee. 1968. *Redeemer nation, the idea of America's millennial role*. Chicago: University of Chicago Press.

Unschuld, Paul U. 1979. *Medical ethics in Imperial China, a study in historical anthropology*. Berkeley: University of California Press.

Valverde, Mariana. 1991. *The age of soap and water: Moral reform in English Canada, 1885–1925*. Toronto: McClelland and Stewart Inc.

Varg, Paul A. 1958. *Missionaries, Chinese and diplomats: The American Protestant missionary movement in China, 1890–1952*. Princeton: Princeton University Press.

————. 1980. *The making of a myth: The United States and China 1897–1912*. Westport: Greenwood Press, 1980.

Walsh, Mary Roth. 1977. *Doctors Wanted: No Women Need Apply, Sexual Barriers in the Medical Profession 1835–1975*. New Haven: Yale University Press.

Weinstein, Fred. 1990. *History and theory after the fall, an essay on interpretation*. Chicago: University of Chicago Press.

Wentworth, Phoebe White and Angie Mills. 1997. *Fair is the Name: The Story of the Shanghai American School, 1912–1950*. Shanghai: Shanghai American School Association.

Woloch, Nancy. 1984. *Women and the American experience*. New York: Knopf.

Women's Division, Board of Global Ministries. 1986. *They went out not knowing: An encyclopedia of one hundred women in mission*. New York: Women's Division, Board of Global Ministries, United Methodist Church.

Articles

Andrews, Bridie J. 1997. Tuberculosis and the assimilation of germ theory in China, 1895–1937. *Journal of the American Medical Association* 52.

Bates, M. Searle. 1974. The theology of American missionaries in China, 1900–1950. In *Missionary enterprise*, edited by John King Fairbank, 135–58.

Beaver, R. Pierce. 1971. Laura Askew Haygood. In *Notable American women 1607–1950: A biographical dictionary*, vol. 2, edited by Edward T. James and Janet Wilson James. Cambridge: Harvard University Press, Belknap Press, 167-69.

Brouwer, Ruth Compton. 1989. Opening doors through social service: Aspects of women's work in the Canadian Presbyterian Mission in Central India, 1877–1914. In *Women's work for women, missionaries and social change in Asia*, edited by Leslie A. Flemming, 11–34.

Brown, Earl Kent. 1974. Archetypes and stereotypes: Church women in the 19th century. *Religion in Life* 43:325–36.

————. 1980. Women in church history: Stereotypes, archtypes and operational modalities. *Methodist History* 18:109–32.

————. 1981. Women of the word: Selected leadership roles of women in Mr. Wesley's Methodism. In *Women in new worlds*, edited by Keller, Queens, and Thomas, 1:69–87.

Brumberg, Joan Jacobs. 1982. Zenanas and girlless villages: The ethnology of American evangelical women, 1870–1910. *Journal of American History* 69:347–71.

Brumberg, Joan Jacobs, and Nancy Tomes. 1982. Women in the professions: A research agenda for American historians. *Reviews in American History* 10:275–96.

Burkhart, Geoffrey. 1989. Danish women missionaries: Personal accounts of work with South Indian women. In *Women's work for women*, edited by Leslie A. Flemming, 59–87.

Carwardine, Richard. 1972. The second great awakening in the urban centers: An examination of Methodism and new measures. *Journal of American History*. 327–40.

Chow, Rey. 1991. Violence in the other country: China as crisis, spectacle, and woman. In *Third world women*, edited by Mohanty, Talpade, and Torreo, 81–100.

Chu, Samuel C. 1980. The New Life Movement before the Sino-Japanese conflict: A reflection of Kuomintang limitations in thought and action. In *China at the crossroads: Nationalists and Communists, 1927–1949*, edited by F. Gilbert Chan. Boulder, CO: Westview Press.

Costigliola, Frank. 1997. The nuclear family: Tropes of gender and pathology in the Western Alliance. *Diplomatic History* 21:2, 163–83.

Cott, Nancy F. 1975. Young women in the second great awakening. *Feminist Studies* 2:15–29.

Croizer, Ralph C. 1973. Traditional medicine as a basis for Chinese medical practice. In *Medicine and public health in the People's Republic of China*, edited by Joseph R. Quinn. Bethesda, MD: National Institute of Health.

Dodson, Jualynne. 1981. Nineteenth-century A. M. E. preaching women: Cutting edge of women's inclusion in church polity. In *Women in new worlds*, edited by Keller, Queens, and Thomas, 1:276–92.

Finke, Roger, and Stark, Rodney. 1989. How the upstart sects won America: 1776–1850. *Journal for the Scientific Study of Religion* 28:27–44.

Flemming, Leslie A. 1989. New models, new roles: U.S. Presbyterian women missionaries and social change in North India, 1870–1910. In *Women's work for women*, edited by Leslie A. Flemming, 35–58.

————. 1992. A new humanity, American missionaries' ideals for women in North India, 1870–1930. In *Western women and Imperialism*, edited by Chaudhuri and Strobel, 191–206.

Garrett, Shirley S. 1974. Why they stayed: American church politics and Chinese Nationalism in the twenties. In *The Missionary enterprise in China and America*, edited by John King Fairbank.

————. 1982. Sister's all: feminism and the American women's missionary movement. *Missionary ideologies in the Imperialist era: 1880–1920*, edited by Torben Christensen and William R. Hutchison. Denmark: Christensen Boytrykkeri, Bogtrykkergarden a-s, Struer, 231–30.

Gifford, Carolyn DeSwarte. 1985. Sisterhoods of service and reform: organized Methodist women in the late nineteenth century. *Methodist History* 23:2, 15–30.

Hardesty, Nancy. 1981. Minister as prophet? or as mother?: Two nineteenth-century models. *Women in new worlds*, edited by Keller, Queens, and Thomas, 1:88–101.

Hatch, Nathan, O. 1993. The puzzle of American Methodism. *Reflections* (Summer-Fall): 13–20. A bi-annual bulletin of the Yale Divinity School.

Higashi, Sumiko. 1979. Cinderella vs. statistics: The silent movie heroine as a jazz-age working girl. *Woman's being, woman's place*, edited by Mary Kelley, 109–26.

Hoyt, Frederick. 1996. Junk mail is not new: China missionaries used direct marketing. *American Philatelist, The Journal of the American Philatelic Society* (November): 1022–29.

Hunter, Jane. 1989. The home and the world: The missionary message of U.S. domesticity. In *Women's work for women*, edited by Leslie A. Flemming, 159–66.

Huskey, James. 1987. The cosmopolitan connection: Americans and Chinese in Shanghai during the interwar years. *Diplomatic History* 11: 3, 227–50.

Iriye, Akira. 1979. Culture and power: International relations as intercultural relations. *Diplomatic History* 3 (Spring): 3:115–28.

———. 1989. The internationalization of history. *American Historical Review* 94:1–10.

Jordan, Donald. 1980. China's vulnerability to Japanese Imperialism: The anti-Japanese boycott of 1931–1932. In *China at the crossroads: Nationalists and Communists, 1927–1949*, edited by F. Gilbert Chan. Boulder, CO: Westview Press. 91–123.

Kaplan, Amy. 1994. Domesticating foreign policy. *Diplomatic History* (Winter) 18:97–105.

Keller, Rosemary Skinner. 1986. Patterns of laywomen's leadership in twentieth-century Protestantism. In *Women and religion in America*, Vol. 3, edited by Rosemary Skinner Keller. San Francisco: Harper & Row, 269–70.

Kelman, Herbert C. 1965. Social-psychological approaches to the study of international relations: The question of relevance. In *International behavior: A social-psychological analysis*, edited by Herbert C. Kelman. New York: Holt, Rinehart and Winston, The Society for the Psychological Study of Social Issues.

Kessler, Lawrence, D. 1990. Hands across the sea: Foreign missions and home support. In *United States attitudes and policies toward China*, edited by Patricia Neils, 78–96.

King, Marjorie. 1989. Exporting femininity, not feminism: Nineteenth-century U.S. missionary women's efforts to emancipate Chinese women. In *Women's work for women*, edited by Leslie A. Flemming, 117–36.

———. 1990. Ida Pruitt, heir and critic of American missionary reform efforts in China. In *United States attitudes and policies toward China*, edited by Patricia Neils, 133–40.

Leffler, Melvyn P. 1995. New approaches, old interpretations, and prospective reconfigurations. *Diplomatic History* 19:2, 173–96.

Lodwick, Kathleen. 1990. Hainan for the homefolk: Images of the island in the missionary and secular presses. In *United States attitudes and policies toward China*, edited by Patricia Neils, 97–110.

Lytle, Mark H. 1996. Environmental approach to diplomatic history. *Diplomatic History* 20:2, 269–300.

McEnaney, Laura. 1994. He-Men and Christian Mothers: The America First Movement and the Gendered Meanings of Patriotism and Isolationism. *Diplomatic History* 18, 47–58.

Merish, Lori. 1993. "The hand of refined taste" in the frontier landscape: Caroline Kirkland's "A new home, who'll follow?" and the feminization of American consumerism. *American Quarterly* 45,4 (December): 485–523.

Rabe, Valentine. 1974. Evangelical logistics: Mission support and resources to 1920. In *Missionary enterprise*, edited by John King Fairbank, 56–90.

Rawlinson, John L. 1990. Frank Rawlinson, China missionary, 1902–1937, veteran deputationist. In *United States attitudes and policies toward China*, edited by Patricia Neils, 111–32.

Rupp, Leila J. 1994. Constructing internationalism: The case of transnational women's organizations, 1888–1945. *The American Historical Review* 99:5, 1571–1600.

Russo, Ann. 1991. We cannot live without our lives: white women, antiracism, and feminism. In *Third world women*, edited by Mohanty, Talpade, and Torres, 297–313.

Selmon, Bertha, M.D. 1945. Pioneer women in medicine: Early service in mission. *Medical Women's Journal* (April): 54.

———. 1947. Pioneer women in medicine, early service in missions. *Medical Woman's Journal* (April): 51–57.

Stapleton, Carolyn. 1983. Belle Harris Bennett: Model for holistic Christianity. *Methodist History* 21:131–42.

Tucker, Sara W. 1989. A mission for change in China: The Hackett Women's Medical Center of Canton, China, 1900–1930. In *Women's work for women*, edited by Leslie A. Flemming, 137–58.

Welter, Barbara. 1966. The cult of true womanhood, 1820–1860. *American Quarterly* 18:151–74.

———. 1976a. Coming of age in America: The American girl in the nineteenth century. In *Dimity convictions: The American woman in the nineteenth century*. Athens: Ohio University Press, 3–21.

———. 1976b. The feminization of American religion: 1800–1860. *Dimity convictions*, 83–102.

———. 1978. She hath done what she could: Protestant women's missionary careers in nineteenth-century America. *American Quarterly* 30:624–38.

Index

Numbers in **boldface** indicate illustrations